Manual of
PEDIATRIC CARDIAC INTENSIVE CARE

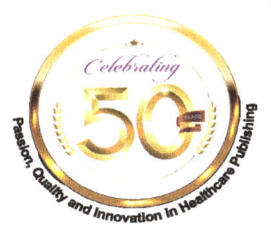

Disclaimer

Every effort has been made to check and verify the drug dosages and the methods of procedure according to the standards accepted at the time of publication. The ultimate responsibility lies with prescribing physicians, based on their professional experience and knowledge of the patient. In no case can the institution with which the author is affiliated and the contributors or the publisher be held responsible for the views expressed in this book. In case of any errors, please notify the author.

Manual of
PEDIATRIC CARDIAC INTENSIVE CARE

SECOND EDITION

Editor
Prashant Shah
MBBS MS DNB Cardiothoracic Surgery(Gold Medal)

Director, Chief Consultant and Pediatric Cardiac Surgeon
Child Heart International, Chennai
Visiting Senior Consultant
Sooriya Hospital, Kanchi Kamakoti Childs Trust Hospital
Chennai, Tamil Nadu, India

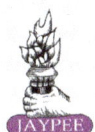

JAYPEE BROTHERS MEDICAL PUBLISHERS
The Health Sciences Publisher
New Delhi | London

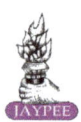

Jaypee Brothers Medical Publishers (P) Ltd

Headquarters
Jaypee Brothers Medical Publishers (P) Ltd
4838/24, Ansari Road, Daryaganj
New Delhi 110 002, India
Phone: +91-11-43574357
Fax: +91-11-43574314
E-mail: jaypee@jaypeebrothers.com

Overseas Office
JP Medical Ltd
83 Victoria Street, London
SW1H 0HW (UK)
Phone: +44 20 3170 8910
Fax: +44 (0)20 3008 6180
E-mail: info@jpmedpub.com

Website: www.jaypeebrothers.com
Website: www.jaypeedigital.com

© 2020, Jaypee Brothers Medical Publishers

The views and opinions expressed in this book are solely those of the original contributor(s)/author(s) and do not necessarily represent those of editor(s) of the book.

All rights reserved. No part of this publication may be reproduced, stored or transmitted in any form or by any means, electronic, mechanical, photocopying, recording or otherwise, without the prior permission in writing of the publishers.

All brand names and product names used in this book are trade names, service marks, trademarks or registered trademarks of their respective owners. The publisher is not associated with any product or vendor mentioned in this book.

Medical knowledge and practice change constantly. This book is designed to provide accurate, authoritative information about the subject matter in question. However, readers are advised to check the most current information available on procedures included and check information from the manufacturer of each product to be administered, to verify the recommended dose, formula, method and duration of administration, adverse effects and contraindications. It is the responsibility of the practitioner to take all appropriate safety precautions. Neither the publisher nor the author(s)/editor(s) assume any liability for any injury and/or damage to persons or property arising from or related to use of material in this book.

This book is sold on the understanding that the publisher is not engaged in providing professional medical services. If such advice or services are required, the services of a competent medical professional should be sought.

Every effort has been made where necessary to contact holders of copyright to obtain permission to reproduce copyright material. If any have been inadvertently overlooked, the publisher will be pleased to make the necessary arrangements at the first opportunity. The **CD/DVD-ROM** (if any) provided in the sealed envelope with this book is complimentary and free of cost. **Not meant for sale.**

Inquiries for bulk sales may be solicited at: jaypee@jaypeebrothers.com

Manual of Pediatric Cardiac Intensive Care
First Edition: 2013
Second Edition: **2020**
ISBN: 978-93-5270-268-8

Dedication

*Second edition is dedicated to
all children with congenital heart defects.*

*My teachers who have taught me how to lead,
my Guruji for his continuous guidance.*

CONTRIBUTORS

Ajith Sunny
MBBS MD PDCC
Consultant Cardiac Anesthesiologist
Department of Cardiac Surgery
MIOT Hospital
Chennai, Tamil Nadu, India

Amit Mishra
MBBS MS MCh FPCS FPCSF
Professor
Department of Pediatric Cardiac Surgery
UN Mehta Institute of Cardiology and Research Centre
Ahmedabad, Gujarat, India

G Selvakumar
MBBS MD FNB
Consultant and Head
Department of Pediatric Cardiac Intensive Care
Madras Medical Mission
Chennai, Tamil Nadu, India

Harun Ramasami
MBBS MS MCh(Cardiac Surgery)
Consultant Pediatric Cardiac Surgeon
Child Heart International
Chennai, Tamil Nadu, India

K Mahalaxmi BS
Physician Assistant Intensive Care Unit
Pediatric Cardiac Intensive Care Unit
Kauvery Hospital
Chennai, Tamil Nadu, India

Kamlesh Tailor
MBBS MD FNB
Chief Consultant
Pediatric Cardiac Intensivist and Anesthesiologist
Kokilaben Dhirubhai Ambani Hospital
Mumbai, Maharashtra, India

Karthik Surya
MBBS DNB(Pediatrics) FNB(Pediatric Cardiology)
Consultant Pediatric Cardiologist
Child Heart International, Chennai
Visiting Consultant
Sooriya Hospital, Kanchi Kamakoti Childs Trust Hospital
Chennai, Tamil Nadu, India

Lakshmi M MBBS MD(Pediatrics)
Consultant Pediatric Cardiac Intensivist
Kauvery Hospital
Chennai, Tamil Nadu, India

M Gokulakrishnan MD PDCC MBA
Consultant Cardiac Anesthesiologist and Intensivist
MIOT Hospital
Chennai, Tamil Nadu, India

Prabhu Mayesesavan MBBS MD
Consultant Pediatric Cardiac Anesthesiologist
Chettinad Health City
Chennai, Tamil Nadu, India

Prashant Prasanna Bhaskar
MBBS MD DM(Cardiac Anesthesia)
Senior Consultant and Pediatric Cardiac Anesthetist
Child Heart International
Chennai, Tamil Nadu, India

Prashant Shah MBBS MS DNB
Cardiothoracic Surgery(Gold Medal)
Director, Chief Consultant and Pediatric Cardiac Surgeon
Child Heart International, Chennai
Visiting Senior Consultant
Sooriya Hospital, Kanchi Kamakoti Childs Trust Hospital
Chennai, Tamil Nadu, India

R Kokila BSc Nursing
Nurse-in-Charge, Pediatric Cardiac Intensive Care Unit
Child Heart Care
Lifeline Hospital
Chennai, Tamil Nadu, India

Ranjith Karthekeyan
MBBS MD DM(Cardiac Anesthesia)
Chief Cardiac Anesthesiologist
Sri Ramachandra Medical College
Chennai, Tamil Nadu, India

Sachin S Patil
MD FNB MHA
Consultant-in-Charge
Pediatric Cardiac
Intensive Care Unit
Fortis Hospital
Mumbai, Maharashtra, India

Sapna Varma
MBBS MD(Anesthesia)
Chief Cardiac Anesthesiologist
MGM Health Care
Chennai, Tamil Nadu, India

Shrishu Kamath
MBBS DCH DNB(Pediatrics)
SIMS Hospital, Chennai
Consultant Pediatric Cardiac
Intensivist
Child Heart International
Chennai, Tamil Nadu, India

Suryanarayanpillai Hari Prakash
DCH MRCP MRCPCH FPCCM
CCT in Pediatric Intensive Care
Medicine Department of Pediatrics
Mildura Base Hospital
Mildura, Victoria, Australia

Yogesh C Sathe MBBS MD FNB
Consultant Pediatric Cardiologist
Narayana Health
Palwal, Haryana, India

PREFACE TO THE SECOND EDITION

It gives me immense pleasure to write preface for the second edition. First edition was appreciated and widely used in most of the centers in India, who performs pediatric cardiac surgeries.

We have added certain new drugs and protocol which has been evolved on time. Basic format of the book has not been changed though.

I sincerely thank all contributors and readers for their contribution and support to bring this second edition. My special thanks to Jaypee Brothers Medical Publishers and team for excellent work.

Prashant Shah

PREFACE TO THE FIRST EDITION

Pediatric cardiac surgery has emerged as a separate subspecialty in cardiac surgery in this decade. The most important aspect for better outcome of congenital cardiac surgery is Pediatric Cardiac Intensive Care. This is my humble effort to put all protocols that we followed successfully together in the form of a book to help new health centers, staff and trainees. This book is a product of years of experience in pediatric cardiac ICU with inputs from many contributors. This book was written as a record of day-to-day activities in Pediatric Cardiac Intensive Care Unit (PCICU), and it should not be considered as a reference book. In this endeavor, I sincerely thank all the contributors, my staff and teachers. I look forward to any feedback and constructive criticism from users, to which we will give due consideration in the future edition.

Prashant Shah

BOOK REVIEW

The *Manual of Pediatric Cardiac Intensive Care* is an excellent handbook to provide instant bedside reference in day-to-day practical management of the cardiac patients in intensive care. It is well laid out, easy to reference and pocket-sized, full of practical information on clinical management as well as educational material on common cardiac conditions. It is designed for surgical, cardiology and intensive care trainees as well as nursing staff but is also a valuable aide memoir for trainees and consultants alike, including valuable reference data on dosages and infusions. Dr Shah's book is the first of its kind and will be a constant companion to clinicians and nurses looking after these patients in intensive care.

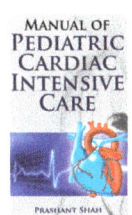

David Barron MD
Senior Consultant and Pediatric Cardiac Surgeon
Department of Pediatric Cardiac Surgery
Birmingham Children's Hospital
Birmingham, UK

ACKNOWLEDGMENTS

I would like to thank everyone who gave me suggestions and constructive criticism, while I prepared this book.

I am particularly grateful to all contributors, for their efforts and invaluable comments on the final draft of the text.

I am thankful to all my team members, for their direct and indirect involvement.

I am especially thankful to Shri Jitendar P Vij (Group Chairman), Mr Ankit Vij (Managing Director), Mr MS Mani (Group President), Ms Chetna Malhotra Vohra (Associate Director—Content Strategy), Ms Pooja Bhandari (Production Head) and Ms Nedup Denka Bhutia (Development Editor) of M/s Jaypee Brothers Medical Publishers, New Delhi, India, for facilitating the editorial process.

CONTENTS

1. Receiving Patient from Operation Theater, Assessment, Preparation and Handing-over Process   **1**
Sachin S Patil, Kamlesh Tailor
- Postoperative Intensive Care Management of the Cardiac Surgical Patient   1
- Ten Commandments for Postoperative Care in the Pediatric Cardiac Intensive Care Unit   1
- Postoperative Care for Cardiac Surgical Patients   2
- Postoperative Handover Proforma   5
- Action Plan on Patient's Arrival in PICU (Secondary Check)   6
- Parents Counseling   7

2. Monitoring Techniques   **8**
Ranjith Karthekeyan
- Monitoring Techniques in the ICU   8
- Electrocardiogram   8
- Arterial Pressure Monitoring   8
- Left Atrial Line   9
- Right Atrial and Central Venous Pressure   10
- Pulmonary Artery Pressure   11
- Cardiac Output and Hemodynamic Variables   11
- Left Atrial Pressure   12
- Respiratory Monitoring   12
- End-Tidal Carbon-Dioxide Monitoring (Capnography)   13

3. Cardiovascular Function and Assessment   **16**
Suryanarayanpillai Hari Prakash, Karthik Surya
- Cardiovascular Management   16
- Special Features of Pediatric Cardiac Management   16
- Assessment of Low Cardiac Output States   17
- Causes of Impaired Cardiac Performance   18
- Low Cardiac Output   20
- Heart Rate and Rhythm   21
- Acceptable Parameters   22
- Volume Status   23
- Cardiac Contractility and Afterload   24
- Left Ventricle and Systemic Vascular Resistance   24
- Right Ventricle and Pulmonary Hypertension   25

4. Respiratory Assessment and Management 27
M Gokulakrishnan
- Respiratory Management 27
- Endotracheal Tubes 27
- Mechanical Ventilators 28
- Ventilator Setting 29
- Management of Children during Mechanical Ventilation 30
- Weaning and Extubation 31

5. Pulmonary Hypertension Crisis and Management 33
Prashant Shah
- Pulmonary Hypertensive Crisis 33

6. Fluid and Electrolyte Management 35
G Selvakumar, Shrishu Kamath, Karthik Surya
- Types of Fluids 37
- Blood Replacement 38
- Hyperkalemia 38
- Hypokalemia 39
- Hypernatremia 40
- Hyponatremia 41
- Magnesium Deficiency 42
- Hypocalcemia 42
- Protocol for Metabolic Acidosis 44
- Treatment 44

7. Mediastinal Bleeding, Cardiac Tamponade and Transfusion Therapy 45
Amit Mishra
- Mediastinal Bleeding and Transfusion Therapy 45
- Blood Products 47
- Packed Red Blood Cells 47
- Platelets 48
- Fresh Frozen Plasma 48
- Cryoprecipitate 49
- Human Albumin Solutions 50
- Cardiac Tamponade 51

8. Capillary Leak Syndrome 52
Prashant Shah

9. Cardiac Arrhythmias 54
Karthik Surya, Yogesh C Sathe
- Common Types and Causes of Arrhythmias 54
- General Approach to ECG 55

Contents **xix**

- Sinus Bradycardia 55
- Sinus Arrhythmia 56
- Supraventricular Tachycardia 56
- Atrial Flutter 57
- Atrial Fibrillation 58
- Junctional Ectopic Tachycardia/His Bundle Tachycardia 58
- Wolff-Parkinson-White Syndrome 59
- Ventricular Premature Beats 59
- Ventricular Tachycardia 60
- Ventricular Fibrillation 60
- First-degree Heart Block 61
- Second-degree Heart Block 61
- Third-degree Heart Block 63

10. Care of the Patient with a Pacemaker 64
Yogesh C Sathe, Harun Ramasami
- Pacemakers 64
- Basic Understanding of Different Pacing Modes 66
- Patient Management 69

11. Chest Drain: Care, Insertion and Removal 70
Amit Mishra
- Chest Tubes: Care, Insertion and Removal 70
- Management of Tubes 70
- Removal of Tubes 70
- Insertion of Intercostal Catheters 71
- Pleural Fluid Aspiration 73

12. Feeding and Nutrition 75
Shrishu Kamath, Lakshmi M

13. Postoperative Pulmonary Subsystem Issues and Management 79
Sachin S Patil, Ajith Sunny
- Postoperative Pulmonary Subsystem Problems: Upper Airways Obstructions 79
- Management 79
- Reintubation 79
- Phrenic Nerve Lesions 80
- Pneumothorax 80
- Hypoxia and Its Management 81
- Pleural Effusion 81
- Chylothorax 81
- Bronchospasm (Wheeze) 83

14. Postoperative Gastrointestinal Issues 84
Prashant Shah
- Paralytic Ileus 84
- Stress Ulcers 84
- Icterus 84
- Necrotizing Enterocolitis 85
- Gastrointestinal Bleeding 85

15. Postoperative Central Nervous System Issues 86
Shrishu Kamath, Lakshmi M
- Protocol for Seizures in Infants and Children 86

16. Postoperative Renal Issues and Peritoneal Dialysis 88
Prashant Shah
- Renal System and Peritoneal Dialysis 88
- Peritoneal Dialysis 89

17. Pain Management (Sedation and Analgesia) 91
Sapna Varma, M Gokulakrishnan
- Properties of an Ideal Sedative 91
- Indications 91
- Sedatives 92
- Dexmedetomidine: Newer Sedative 92
- Analgesics 93
- Muscle Relaxants 94
- Nondepolarizing Muscle Relaxants 94
- Rocuronium 95
- Atracurium 95

18. Inotropes 96
Prabhu Mayesesavan, Prashant Prasanna Bhaskar
- Dopamine 96
- Epinephrine 96
- Norepinephrine 97
- Dobutamine 97
- Isoproterenol 98
- Bipyridines (Phosphodiesterase Inhibitors) 98
- Vasodilators 99
- Vasoconstrictor 100
- Levosimendan (Inodilator) 101

19. Postoperative Anticoagulation 103
Prashant Shah
- Indication 103
- Agents Used 103
- Warfarin 103

20. Routine General Care 105
K Mahalaxmi, R Kokila
- Oral Hygiene 105
- Bladder Care 105
- Bowel Care 105
- Nasogastric Tube and Gastric Aspiration 106
- Care of Urinary Catheter 106
- Temperature 106
- Protocol for Hyperthermia 106
- Routine Care of Oral or Nasal Endotracheal Tube 107
- Care of Eyes 108
- Skin Care 108
- Tracheostomy Care 108
- Physiotherapy and Endotracheal Suction 110
- Endotracheal Suctioning 112
- Preparing for ET Suction 112

21. Infection Issues and Antimicrobials 114
Prashant Shah, Amit Mishra
- Infection Issues 114
- Sepsis 114
- Prevention 115
- Antibiotics 115
- Recommended Antimicrobial Agents against Selected Organisms 117

22. Postpericardiotomy Syndrome 120
Prashant Shah
- Lab Investigations 121
- Treatment 121

23. Congenital Heart Defect with Specific Issue 122
Prashant Shah, Kamlesh Tailor
- Blalock-Taussig Shunt 122
- Bi-directional Glenn Shunt 124
- Pulmonary Artery Banding 126
- Fontan Procedure 127
- Atrial Septal Defect 128
- Ventricular Septal Defect 129
- Atrioventricular Canal Defect 130
- Total Anomalous Pulmonary Venous Connection 131
- Tetralogy of Fallot 132
- Truncus Arteriosus 134
- Coarctation of Aorta 135
- Aortic Stenosis 136

- Transposition of Great Arteries 137
- Anomalous Left Coronary Artery from Pulmonary Artery 139
- Hypoplastic Left Heart Syndrome 140
- Balancing Shunts Preoperatively 143
- Postoperative Management of Norwood Stage 1 144
- Balancing Shunts Postoperatively 144

APPENDICES

Appendix 1: Drug, Dilution, Administration and Dose 147

- Drug Dosages in Pediatric Cardiac Intensive Care Unit 147
- Inotropes 147
- Chronotropes 148
- Vasodilators 148
- Narcotics 149
- Muscle Relaxants 149
- Loop Diuretics 150
- Osmotic Diuretics 150
- Anticonvulsants 151
- Electrolytes 151
- Bronchodilators 152
- Coagulants 152
- Anticoagulants 153
- Steroids 153
- Antiarrhythmics 154
- Antihypertensives 155
- Antacids 155
- Sedatives 156
- Antiemetics 156
- Reversal Drugs 156
- Antipyretics 156
- Analgesics 157
- Pulmonary Hypertension 157
- Hematinics 157
- Miscellaneous 157
- Laxatives 158
- Nebulizing Agents 158
- Antibiotics Aminoglycosides 159
- Cephalosporines 159
- Fluoroquinolones 160
- Penicillin Group 160
- Antifungal 160
- Miscellaneous 161

Appendix 2: Flowcharts   **162**
Suryanarayanpillai Hari Prakash

Appendix 3: Guidelines for Endotracheal Suction   **166**
Prabhu Mayakesavan
- Guidelines for Endotracheal Suction PICU (Royal Liverpool Children's NHS Trust)   166

Appendix 4: Responsibilities of the Bedside Nurse when Chest Closing or Opening   **168**
K Mahalaxmi, R Kokila
- Before the Procedure   168
- During the Procedure   168
- After the Procedure   169

Index   *171*

Chapter 1

Receiving Patient from Operation Theater, Assessment, Preparation and Handing-over Process

Sachin S Patil, Kamlesh Tailor

POSTOPERATIVE INTENSIVE CARE MANAGEMENT OF THE CARDIAC SURGICAL PATIENT

A multidisciplinary team approach with coordination between multiple services (cardiac surgeon, cardiologist, intensivist, anesthesiologist, pediatrician, respiratory therapist, cardiac critical care-trained nurse) is the key to a successful outcome in the postoperative intensive care management of any cardiac surgical patient, undergoing a palliative or corrective procedure for a congenital heart defect.

The surgical procedure comprises anesthetic induction, prebypass period, and the cardiopulmonary bypass (CPB) and postbypass period.

TEN COMMANDMENTS FOR POSTOPERATIVE CARE IN THE PEDIATRIC CARDIAC INTENSIVE CARE UNIT (PCICU)

- Constant vigil is the key to a successful outcome. The PCICU is never like an unmanned level crossing.
- Multidisciplinary approach in providing quality care services is mandatory.
- Frequent clinical monitoring is as vital as high tech bedside monitors.
- Sudden untoward events (e.g. cardiac arrest) necessitating prompt action, though rare, is not uncommon.
- Problems should be anticipated and complications prevented by instituting appropriate therapy.
- There is a cause for everything, and these causes should be identified for timely management.
- Two management parameters should not be altered at the same time.
- There should be no hesitation in calling seniors for assistance in difficult situations.

- Establishment of standard protocols in management and refinement of communication skills should be adhered to for maintaining continuity of care. Seniors should be consulted when change is contemplated.
- Common things should be thought about first.

POSTOPERATIVE CARE FOR CARDIAC SURGICAL PATIENTS

Inadequate postoperative care can nullify the benefits of a meticulously carried out complex cardiac repair and result in morbidity or even mortality.

Effective postoperative care includes:
- Continuous monitoring of functions of cardiac hemodynamic, pulmonary and other vital organs such as liver, kidney and central nervous system (CNS).
- Prompt appropriate corrective measures to restore normal function when deviations from normal are identified.

Checklist of Items that should be Always Available in PCICU

- Central O_2 delivery, suction line with optimal functioning.
- Airways, laryngoscope, endotracheal (ET) tubes, suction catheters and ventilator.
- Defibrillator with appropriately sized pediatric paddles and cardiac monitors.
- Ambu bag with masks for various age groups, including neonates.
- Intravenous access tray including central line.
- Peritoneal dialysis (PD) tray with catheter and instruments.
- Chest tubes for decompression of pneumothorax/draining pleural effusions.
- Cardiac pacemakers.
- Syringe pumps and infusion pumps.
- Nasogastric (NG) tubes.
- Urine collection system with Foley's catheters.
- Syringes, medicuts, three ways, stop cocks, suction catheters, etc.
- All emergency medications (*see* Appendix 1).
- Stethoscope for individual patients.
- Thermometer.

Preparation to be Done before Receiving Patient in PCICU

- Prepare case sheet, ICU sheet.
- Calculate inotropes according to patient's weight.

- Check ventilators, syringe pump, infusion pump, defibrillator, pacing cables and pacemaker.
- Check air, O_2, suction line.
- Check that emergency drugs are loaded, and that the intubation and extubation tray checks are done.
- Keep drainage bottle ready.
- Prepare mentally for the particular case and read or discuss with team or senior staff.

Transferring Patient from Operating Room

- Transfer of the pediatric cardiac surgical patient from the operating room to the ICU is a critical phase during which problems such as displacement of the endotracheal tube, intravenous lines, alteration in drug infusion rates or hypothermia from exposure to ambient temperature may occur leading to sudden deterioration.
- Several measures should be taken to ensure a well-organized transfer from the operating room.
    - The child should be hemodynamically stable before transfer.
    - Confirm the absence of active bleeding.
    - All catheters and tubes must be sutured and secured to the skin and reinforced with tape. If nasotracheal tube is used, it should be secured to the upper lip.
    - Continuous monitoring of the electrocardiogram (ECG), arterial blood pressure and pulse-oximeter oxygen saturations should be ensured by checking that the transport monitor has a battery back-up. At no point of time the vital signs should be off-line.
    - All medication should be infused using portable infusion control devices whose battery function is ensured before transfer.
    - Adequate volume of blood products should be available during transport.
    - Emergency drugs tray to be carried with the child.
    - Connect the pacing wires to the pacemaker in demand mode before shifting. If the child is pacemaker dependent, ensure that the pacemaker battery is new and the pacing wires are properly secured with tape.
    - Oxygen cylinder should be full and the flow-meter functioning with a working Ambu bag appropriate for the size of the child.
    - The child should be shifted from the operation table to the PCICU bed with the command for '1-2-3-shift.'
    - In case the chest is kept open strict aseptic precautions should be taken during the transfer.

- If the child is shifted on a bed warmer then the warmer should be switched on at least 30 minutes prior to shifting the child on it to prevent hypothermia.
- The PCICU should be aware in advance about the surgery performed, ventilatory settings required, inotropes dosages and the intracardiac lines that have been place.

Arrival of Patient to PCICU (Preliminary Check)

- Follow a standard acceptance protocol to ensure a safe transition to the ICU. An individual well versed in pediatric intensive care who is an expert in intubation, line insertion, pharmacologic intervention and monitoring techniques should supervise the patient's arrival in the PCICU.
- Airway/ventilator:
  - Check breathing sounds by auscultation and chest wall movement during manual and mechanical ventilation.
  - Select initial ventilator settings:
    - FiO_2 = according to requirements.
    - Tidal volume = 10–15 mL/kg.
    - Peak pressure <25 cm H_2O.
    - Positive end-expiratory pressure (PEEP) = 2–5 cm H_2O.
    - Respiratory rate:
      - Newborn: 30–40/min.
      - Infant: 20–30/min.
      - Older than 1 year: 18–28/min.
  - I/E ratio = 1:2 (use a 1:1 ratio in neonates and young infants, who benefit from a longer inspiratory phase to minimize airway resistance).
- Vital signs:
  - Confirm rate, rhythm and ECG morphology using a portable monitor and then connect the leads to the bedside monitor.
  - Check blood pressure manually by auscultation or by Doppler method.
  - Check the femoral arterial pulse; if these parameters are satisfactory, connect the arterial line to the calibrated bedside monitor and correlate side play with manual readings.
  - Connect intracardiac line to a calibrated bedside monitor and record the reading. Consider the air filter for both intracardiac and peripheral IV line in small infants.
  - Record the temperature.

- Observe the initial amount of chest tube drainage in the collection chamber and examine the amount of blood within the chest tube.
- Physical examination:
  - Auscultate for bilateral breath sound.
  - Examine the extremities for pulse, capillary refill and temperature.
  - Check all intracardiac lines, chest tubes and pacing electrodes for security.
  - Check for pupil reaction.
- The anesthesia and surgical teams should give a comprehensive report to the ICU physician and nursing staff.
- Write postoperative order for fluids and drug therapy.
- Perform supine chest X-ray to know the ET tube position, lung fields, location of intracardiac lines and NG tube position.

The Handover Process

- The handover begins once the child is shifted from the OT to the PCICU, the ventilator is connected, settings are checked, monitors are attached and the bed is parked.
- The handover is given by the anesthesiologist conducting the case to the PCICU team.
- The following personnel are present during the handover:
  - Anesthesiologist shifting the child.
  - Consultant intensivist on day/night (if the patient is shifted after 6 pm) call.
  - Pediatric registrar on duty.
  - Operating surgeon.
  - Nurse taking charge of the patient.
  - Nursing team leader for that shift.
- The handover is started by the anesthesiologist as per the pocket guide.
- The pediatric registrar starts writing the points discussed in a separate sheet provided on similar lines to those mentioned in the bedside writing pad.
- There are no interruptions from the team till the handover is complete.
- Questions are asked only after completion of handover, i.e. once the anesthesiologist finishes his/her handover.

POSTOPERATIVE HANDOVER PROFORMA OT to PCICU

- Patient details:
  - Name, age, sex, weight, Umique Health Identification (UHID) No.

- Preoperative status.
- Planned and performed operation.
- Has the anesthesiologist discussed:
    - Issues during induction.
    - ETT size, route, fixed at.
    - Concerns regarding airway management.
    - Concerns regarding invasive lines.
    - Duration: CPB, ACC, TCA.
    - Concerns regarding weaning from CPB.
    - HR/ ABP/ CVP/ LA/ PA/ SpO_2/ PIP.
    - Modified ultrafiltration and post-MUF hematocrit.
    - Inotropes.
    - Rhythm and pacemaker settings.
    - TEE/epicardial echo findings.
    - Blood products transfused/remaining.
    - Last antibiotic dose.
- Has the surgeon discussed:
    - Surgery performed.
    - Issues with the procedure.
    - Risk of further bleeding and transfusions required.
    - Concerns regarding postoperative recovery.
    - Plan for ventilation.
    - Gauze count or number if chest kept open.
- Has the anesthesiologist, surgeon, intensivist summarized: "all in agreement" and nurses clear about:
    - Plan for next 12–24 hours: Volume/ionotropes/sedation.
    - Anticipated problems.
    - Labs/imaging over next 24 hours.
- Questions and answers.

ACTION PLAN ON PATIENT'S ARRIVAL IN PICU (Secondary Check)

Confirm the following from the preliminary check after the patient settles down in the PCICU and the handover process is complete

- ECG leads in correct position—ascertain rate and rhythm.
- Central monitoring lines connected and values noted—arterial, left/right atrial (arterial BP, CVP).
- Ventilator connections done, leak checked and confirm ventilator settings.
- Chest drain tubes connected to suction bottles (10–20 cm H_2O) check for air leaks and milk the drains to ensure that tubes are clear.
- Urinary catheter connected to urinary bag.
- Pacing wires connected to pacemaker with mode and settings checked.

- Insert nasogastric tube, if patient is on ventilator and otherwise of ordered.
- Check on clinical profile. Check on level of sensorium, chest drainage, dressing for soaking, peripheries for level of warmth, capillary refill time for perfusion, and auscultate both chest and abdomen for liver and fluid.
- Check core temperature.
- Check on orders about fluid therapy, analgesics, sedatives, diuretics, antibiotics, inotropes, etc.
- Investigations:
  - Immediate chest X-ray and, if indicated, 4 hours later; otherwise after 24 hours.
  - Arterial blood gases, electrolytes, Na^+, K^+, Ca^{2+}, Mg^{2+}.
  - ECG—all 12 leads for open heart repairs.
  - *Hematological:* Hb, HCT, TC, DC, ESR.
  - Activated partial thromboplastin time (APTT)/prothrombin time (PT)/international normalized ratio (INR).
  - ACT (if increased drainage).
  - *Biochemical:* Liver function tests, serum bilirubin, serum glutamic oxaloacetic transaminase (SGOT), serum glutamic oxaloacetic transaminase (SGPT) and blood glucose, protein, albumin.
  - *Renal:* Blood urea and serum creatinine.
  - CPK-MB if anomalous left coronary artery from pulmonary artery (ALCAPA), switch procedure (0h, 4h, 12h and 1 day).

PARENTS COUNSELING

Once the child has stabilized in the PCICU and the operating surgeon has spoken to the parents; they should be encouraged to see their child. During this first visit, they should be explained about the expected course of management (based on the cardiac lesion) in regards to weaning from ventilation, concerns about analgesia, sedation and awakening, probable resumption of feeding, and the visiting hours.

Chapter 2

Monitoring Techniques

Ranjith Karthekeyan

MONITORING TECHNIQUES IN THE ICU

- Monitoring is essential to the daily care of ICU patients to optimize patient's hemodynamic and ventilatory status so that the oxygen demand of the tissues is met. Both oxygenation and perfusion monitoring is essential for the implementation of any resuscitation strategy.
- *Noninvasive monitoring:* Electrocardiogram, pulse-oximeter, respiratory rate measurement, non-invasive blood pressure and end tidal carbon dioxide.
- *Invasive monitoring devices:* Central venous pressure, continuous arterial pressure, left atrial pressure, pulmonary artery pressure, cardiac output monitoring and arterial blood gas.

ELECTROCARDIOGRAM (FIG. 2.1)

One of the most useful ways of monitoring critically-ill patients. Continuous ECG display of leads II and V5 permits monitoring for ischemia and dysarrhythmias. Also important in cases of electrolyte disturbances and drug overdoses.

ARTERIAL PRESSURE MONITORING (FIG. 2.2)

Direct arterial pressures can be recorded by inserting a cannula in the radial, femoral or dorsalis pedis artery and connecting it to a zeroed and calibrated transducer which

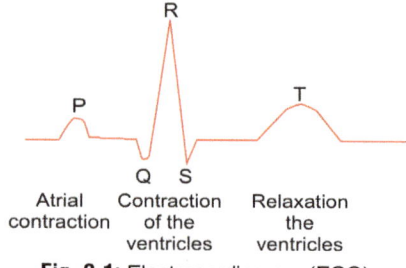

Fig. 2.1: Electrocardiogram (ECG).

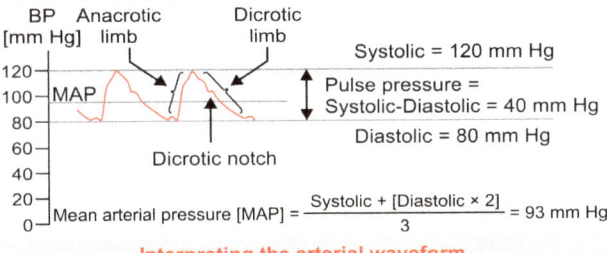

Interpreting the arterial waveform

As pressure falls, the aortic valve closes-signaling the onset of diastole, aortic valve closure produces a characteristic waveform known as the dicrotic notch (see above). As diastole progresses, the pressure falls to its lowest level. The lowest value of the arterial waveform is the diastolic pressure. Normal diastolic pressure ranges between 60 and 90 mm Hg.

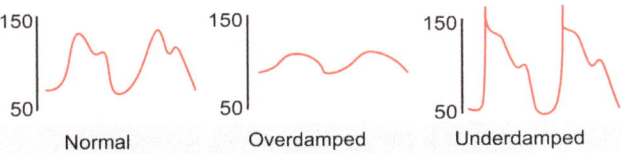

Fig. 2.2: Arterial waveform.

converts pressure energy into electrical. Arterial blood pressure is proportional to cardiac output when peripheral resistance is constant.

The presence of air bubbles, leaks in the system or blocked cannulae can produce an excessively damped trace. The system is said to be optimally damped when the dicrotic notch of the waveform can be readily distinguished and the systolic waveform is not too spiky.

Extreme care is taken to maintain the patency of arterial lines and protect them from inadvertent disconnection. A continuous flush device is used to prevent line thrombosis. Forceful manual flushing is avoided because it damages the vessel and propels air bubbles and small clots retrograde into the aortic arch and up to the brain. A low-pressure alarm is used to bring attention to disconnection, which could result in exsanguination.

These catheters may be a source of sepsis and peripheral emboli, which may cause loss of a finger, toe or even an entire extremity. Attention to distal perfusion is essential. Pulse oximetry may draw attention to impaired peripheral perfusion beyond the catheter.

LEFT ATRIAL (LA) LINE

Left atrial catheters provide valuable information about the status of the left ventricular (LV) volume. They are of particular value in patients with potential right ventricular (RV) dysfunction in whom the central venous pressure (CVP) may have little correlation with left-sided filling pressures. They are mainly used in high-risk cases like anomalous left coronary artery from the pulmonary artery (ALCAPA), arterial switch procedure.

These catheters are potentially very dangerous, because they may introduce air or thromboembolism into the cerebral or systemic circulations.

Note: Keep chest tube till LA line is removed as it might bleed and may require re-exploration.

RIGHT ATRIAL (RA) AND CENTRAL VENOUS PRESSURE (FIG. 2.3)

- CVP catheters can be inserted at different sites but in each case the tip of the catheter should be intrathoracic. Sites used for the insertion of cannulae include the external jugular vein, internal jugular vein (high or low approach), subclavian vein, femoral vein and the antecubital vein. The Seldinger technique is used most commonly.
- The value of the CVP can be obtained using a saline filled manometer, zeroed to the midaxillary line as

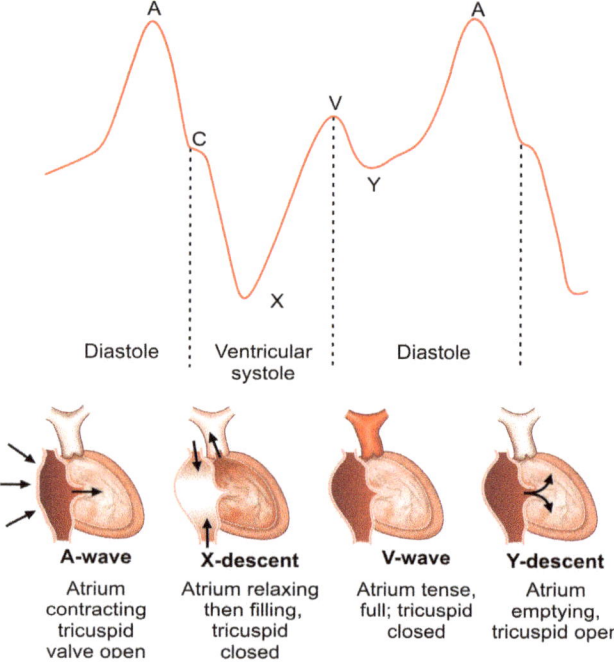

Fig. 2.3: Right atrial (RA) and central venous pressure (CVP).

the reference point, or by using a pressure transducer. Normally CVP ranges between 6 and 12 mm Hg. There can be a discrepancy between CVP and left side heart filling pressures in patient with chronic obstructive airways disease (COAD), pulmonary hypertension or mitral valve disease.

- A-wave—due to atrial contraction. Absent in atrial fibrillation. Enlarged in tricuspid stenosis, pulmonary stenosis and pulmonary hypertension.
- C-wave—due to bulging of tricuspid valve into the right atrium or possibly transmitted pulsations from the carotid artery.
- X-descent—due to atrial relaxation.
- V-wave—due to the rise in atrial pressure before the tricuspid valve opens. Enlarged in tricuspid regurgitation.
- Y-descent—due to atrial emptying as blood enters the ventricle.
- Canon waves—large waves not corresponding to A, V or C-waves. Owing to complete heart block or junctional arrhythmias.

PULMONARY ARTERY (PA) PRESSURE

Pulmonary artery occlusion pressure is used to monitor the left ventricular end diastolic pressures provided the mitral valve is normal. The balloon tipped pulmonary flotation catheter (length 110 cm) is introduced through an insertion sheath (placed in the internal jugular vein or subclavian vein).

Normally the pulmonary artery occlusion pressure (PAOP) varies between 8 and 12 mm Hg. Patients with poor left ventricular function have a PAOP exceeding 18 mm Hg.

Pulmonary artery catheters are extremely useful in the critically-ill patient since not only can PAOP and cardiac output be measured but also the derived parameters, such as systemic and pulmonary vascular resistance and cardiac work, can be used to guide therapy. Clinical applications of these catheters have widened to include oximetry (mixed venous oxygen saturation), pacing and right ventricular ejection fraction.

The main indications for the use of pulmonary artery catheters are poor left ventricular function (due to ischemia, valvular heart disease, cardiomyopathy and aneurysm), sepsis, burns, trauma, acute respiratory distress syndrome (ARDS) and those with major fluid shifts for other reasons.

CARDIAC OUTPUT AND HEMODYNAMIC VARIABLES

Cardiac output can be measured using the Fick principle:
$$\text{Cardiac output (CO)} = VO_2/CaO_2 - CvO_2$$

Where CaO_2 is the arterial oxygen content, CvO_2 is the mixed venous oxygen content and VO_2 is the oxygen consumption.

In practice, a pulmonary artery catheter is used which has a temperature sensor at its end (thermistor tipped). Cold 5% dextrose or 0.9% saline (either 5 or 10 mL) is rapidly injected into the right atrium through the CVP lumen of the catheter and its temperature is automatically sensed at the site of injection. The thermistor at the tip of the catheter within the pulmonary artery is also sensed automatically and compared with that at the CVP injection port. A curve is obtained by the cardiac output computer which plots temperature change with time.

Systemic vascular resistance (SVR) = mean arterial blood pressure – CVP/CO × 80.

Pulmonary vascular resistance (PVR) = mean pulmonary artery pressure – PAOP/CO × 80.

Normal values are 770–1500 and 20–120 dyne.sec/cm^{-5} respectively.

Left ventricular stroke work index (LVSWI) = Stroke volume index × mean arterial pressure × 0.0144.

Normal range is 44–68 g/m^2.

Idea of the adequacy of both supply and tissue uptake can be seen from monitoring the mixed venous oxygen saturation (which can either be performed automatically by some pulmonary artery catheters or by intermittent blood sampling and then measuring oxygen saturation using a co-oximeter).

LEFT ATRIAL PRESSURE

Left atrial catheters provide valuable information about the status of the left ventricular (LV) volume. They are of particular value in patients with potential right ventricular (RV) dysfunction in whom the central venous pressure (CVP) may have little correlation with left-sided filling pressures. They are mainly used in high-risk cases like ALCAPA, arterial switch procedure and total anomalous pulmonary venous connection (TAPVC).

RESPIRATORY MONITORING

- Respiratory rate is monitored electronically as well as manually. Mechanical ventilators have rate and pressure alarms that are activated by apneic events.
- Oxygenation is assessed by ABG analysis and pulse oximetry. Pulse oximetry is dependent on peripheral perfusion. It is beneficial in both intubated and extubated patients.

- Ventilation is monitored by the end-tidal CO_2, which is measured by infrared analysis of the concentration of CO_2 in expired gases. It may also reflect changes in cardiac output and pulmonary blood flow.

END-TIDAL CARBON-DIOXIDE MONITORING (CAPNOGRAPHY)

- End-tidal CO_2 (Pet TCO_2) is the amount of CO_2 in the gas at end exhalation. The value correlates with $PaCO_2$ in normal individuals. The sample gas is usually obtained from a main stream or side stream adaptor, but the adaptor size can increase circuit dead space. The readings can be affected by secretions and moisture.
- It is useful for tracking trends in $PaCO_2$ rather than for predicting exact $PaCO_2$. In adults and children with large tidal volumes and relatively low respiratory rates, the end-tidal gas is entirely alveolar gas, and values reflecting $PaCO_2$ are reliable. It is measured and displayed in a waveform (Figs. 2.3 to 2.6).
- It is a function of four factors: $PaCO_2$, cardiac output, dead space in percent of tidal volume (V_o/V_r) and airway time constants.
- Thus, $PetCO_2$ monitoring can be used to observe adequacy of alveolar ventilation, estimate changes in metabolic output (i.e. CO_2 production), evaluate cardiac output and assess pulmonary perfusion relative to alveolar ventilation (i.e. percent dead space ventilation). The validity of capnography in assessing alveolar ventilation is highest when $PetCO_2$ approximates $PaCO_2$. However, even in healthy persons, the value is 1.5 mm Hg lower than $PaCO_2$ because of the contribution of nonventilating and poorly ventilating lung units to the measured value.
- The disparity between $PaCO_2$ to $PetCO_2$ will increase in the presence of ventilated poorly perfused alveoli

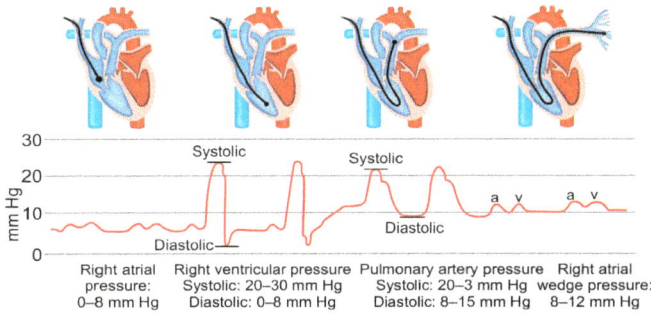

Fig. 2.4: Wave pattern during PA line insertion.

Manual of Pediatric Cardiac Intensive Care

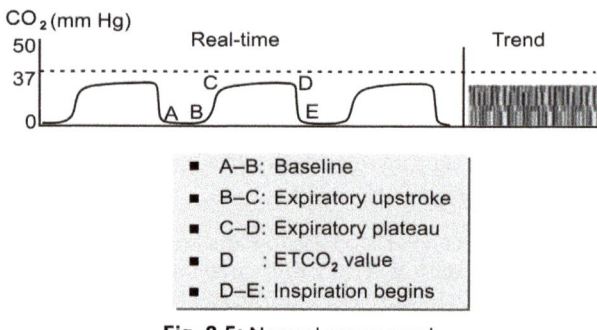

- A–B: Baseline
- B–C: Expiratory upstroke
- C–D: Expiratory plateau
- D : ETCO₂ value
- D–E: Inspiration begins

Fig. 2.5: Normal capnograph.

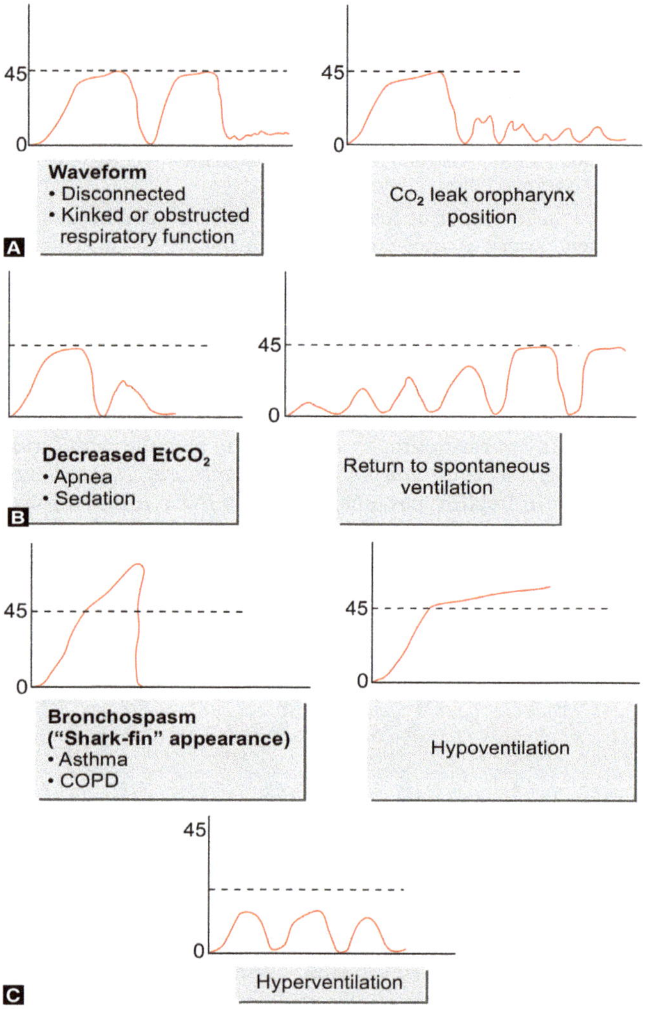

A

Waveform
- Disconnected
- Kinked or obstructed respiratory function

CO₂ leak oropharynx position

B

Decreased EtCO₂
- Apnea
- Sedation

Return to spontaneous ventilation

Bronchospasm ("Shark-fin" appearance)
- Asthma
- COPD

Hypoventilation

C

Hyperventilation

Figs. 2.6A to C: Abnormal capnographs.

(i.e. dead space ventilation) $V_o/V_r = PaCO_2-(PetCO_2/PaCO_2)$. Hence, as dead space increases, $PetCO_2$ underestimates $PaCO_2$, such situations arise during low cardiac output states, increased PVR, excessive PEEP, reduction in pulmonary vascular bed: ARDS, pulmonary emboli, ECMO and CPB. In these situations, capnography is not a measure of alveolar ventilation but a maker of pulmonary perfusion.

- Alternatively, conditions that increase $PaCO_2$ (reduced alveolar ventilation or increase CO_2 production) increase $PetCO_2$ in the presence of constant pulmonary perfusion.
- A fall in $PetCO_2$ with a concomitant decrease in the $PaCO_2$ with a constant gradient reflects either improved alveolar ventilation (Va) or reduced CO_2 production (VCO_2).
- A fall in $PetCO_2$ in the presence of unchanged or increased $PaCO_2$ denotes increased dead space ventilation.
- An increase in $PetCO_2$ with concomitant increase in $PaCO_2$ is consistent with reduced alveolar ventilation or increased VCO_2 (CO_2 production) (e.g. malignant hyperthermia).
- An increase in $PetCO_2$ with an unchanged $PaCO_2$ (i.e. reduced gradient) signifies increased time constants of the airway (resistance or compliance is increased).
- Monitoring of $PetCO_2$ is useful for verification of endotracheal intubation. It can assist in the titration of PEEP by observation of the lowest $PaCO_2$-$PetCO_2$ gradient, indicating that recruitment of alveoli is maximal. Minimizing the gradient may prevent overdistention of alveoli. This is useful in assessing effectiveness of cardiopulmonary resuscitation and cardiac output.
- For all practical purposes, $PetCO_2$ monitoring can be done only in patients with ET tube or tracheostomy in place.
- Changes in $PetCO_2$ must be compared with $PaCO_2$ value to find the cause of the gas exchange derangement.

Chapter 3

Cardiovascular Function and Assessment

Suryanarayanpillai Hari Prakash, Karthik Surya

CARDIOVASCULAR MANAGEMENT

The basic concepts of cardiovascular physiology and the management of cardiovascular derangements after surgery have been elucidated. This section concentrates on the special problems encountered in pediatric patients after cardiac surgery.

SPECIAL FEATURES OF PEDIATRIC CARDIAC MANAGEMENT

- Variable pathology. The nature of the congenital heart defect, the adequacy of the palliative or corrective procedure and any residual pathophysiologic abnormalities must be taken into consideration when selecting a course of management. Some of these factors include:
  - The effects of the congenital defect on the ventricles (hypertrophy or dilatation) and on the pulmonary vascular resistance.
  - Lesions left uncorrected (valve stenosis or insufficiency, small pulmonary arteries, intracardiac shunt).
  - Surgical trauma (suboptimal myocardial protection, ventriculotomy incisions, heart block).
  - The possibility of an inadequate or disrupted surgical repair (thrombosed systemic-to-pulmonary shunts, residual intracardiac shunts, persistent valve stenosis or insufficiency after a valve repair).
- Compensatory mechanisms for impaired cardiac function are more effective in children than in adults, which may mask the extent of cardiac dysfunction. Tachycardia is one of the major compensatory mechanisms to maintain cardiac output following surgery. Significant hypovolemia and poor contractility may be present at normal blood pressure because of increased systemic resistance. Attention to signs of circulatory decompression (impaired perfusion, oliguria and acidosis) is a means of improving cardiac function because the development of hypotension is a late sign of profound decompression.

- Monitoring limitations may also prevent the early detection of cardiovascular decompression. Invasive monitoring to measure the cardiac output directly (Swan-Ganz catheter, PA pressure line and thermistors) is cumbersome, hazardous and is generally avoided except in complex cases. Intracardiac monitoring is usually limited to right atrium (RA) and left atrium (LA) lines:
  - The RA and LA lines provide information on loading conditions of the ventricles; inferences about the status of ventricular function can be made as well, especially after serial volume challenges. Elevated filling pressures suggest the presence of ventricular dysfunction downstream to the measurement.
  - The arterial pulse pressure is the reflection of left ventricular stroke volume and should exceed 20–25 mm Hg in small children. An arterial pulse pressure of less than 15 mm Hg is a sign of low cardiac output.
  - A mixed venous oxygen intracardiac shunt reflects either anemia or a low cardiac output. The SvO_2 is ideally measured using a PA catheter, but in its absence, samples drawn from the RA or CVP line are fairly representative.

ASSESSMENT OF LOW CARDIAC OUTPUT STATES

- Owing to limited monitoring techniques, the assessment of cardiac output must involve a careful patient examination with particular attention paid to peripheral perfusion (skin, color, temperature, pedal pulse, capillary refill), and liver size (to assess RA pressure and fluid status).
- Urine output is usually a reflection of myocardial function. Evidence of oliguria (<1 mL/kg/h) in a child suggests a low output state.
- The development of metabolic acidosis is a reflection of inadequate tissue perfusion, which is irreversible spiral of cardiac decompensation and must be treated aggressively.
- Special care must be taken to normalize the core temperature so that the temperature of the extremities can be used as an index of cardiac function. Measures include use of a heated humidifier in the ventilator circuit, a heating blanket, overhead infrared warmer, and fluid and blood infusion warmers. A core temperature over 39°C reflects a high systemic vascular resistance (SVR) and inability to conduct heat.
- Clinical deterioration should prompt a repeat physical examination. For example, absence of bilateral breath sounds may indicate a pneumothorax; loss of a shunt

murmur may explain increasing cyanosis; reappearance of a ventricular septal defect (VSD) murmur following closure may account for recurrent heart failure.
- Clinical assessment—Table 3.1 is a guide to clinical assessment of cardiac output.

CAUSES OF IMPAIRED CARDIAC PERFORMANCE

The major causes of impaired cardiac performance after open-heart surgery are:
- Hypovolemia:
  - Redistribution.
  - Blood loss.
- Capillary leak, ascites, effusions.
- Myocardial dysfunction—postoperative ischemia (X clamping).
- Residual lesions, e.g. VSD, obstructive lesions.
- Increased afterload—including pulmonary hypertension.
- Abnormalities of heart rate and rhythm:
  - Bradycardia—fixed SV.
  - Tachycardia—filling time.
- Subendocardial perfusion.

TABLE 3.1: Clinical findings in low cardiac output state.

Category	Parameter	Finding/Data
Physical examination		
	Peripheral perfusion	Cool or mottled extremities Diminished peripheral pulses Delayed capillary refill
	Respiratory status	Tachypnea, increased work of breathing grunting flaring retractions
	Cardiac examination	S3 or S4, diminished heart tones, tachycardia or bradycardia
	Other physical examination	Diaphoresis, hepatomegaly, jugular venous distension, increasing cyanosis
	Mental status	Lethargy or irritability
Monitor data		
	Arterial waveform	Diminished pulse pressure, decreased upslope, hypotension, increased variation with respiration
	Atrial filling pressures	Significantly elevated or decreased, lack of 'a' wave

Contd...

Contd...

Category	Parameter	Finding/Data
	ECG	Nonsinus rhythm tachycardia, bradycardia, ST-segment depression or elevation, lack of HR variability
	End-tidal CO_2	Decrease in $ETCO_2$ large end-tidal to arterial CO_2 difference
	Temperature	Increased core-to-periphery temperature gradient (>5°C core to toe)
	Mixed venous (PA) or central venous (SVC) oxygen saturation	Low SvO_2 or $ScVO_2$ <50%
	Near-infrared spectroscopy regional oxygen saturation	Low cerebral rSO_2 <50%
Laboratory and radiographic date		
	Serum lactate	Increasing or persistently elevated over 2 mmol/L
	Calculated base deficit	Increasing or >5 mEq/L
	BNP	Elevated above 100 pg/mL and increasing
	Troponin-I	Elevated above 0.15 ng/mL and increasing
	Chest radiograph	Cardiomegaly, pulmonary edema or paucity of lung vascular markings
	Renal function	Elevated BUN and creatinine Poor urine output <0.5 mL/kg/hr
Echocardiography		
	LV ejection fraction or shortening fraction, dilated LV	Decreased (EF <50% or SF <35%)
Calculated cardiac index		
	Thermodilution, lithium dilution, pulse contour analysis, echocardiographic by VTI method	2.0 L/min/m^2

(S3-S4: third and fourth heart sounds; ETCO: end-eidal carbon dioxide; PA: pulmonary artery; SVC: superior vena cava; SvO: mixed venous oxygen saturation; $ScvO_2$: mixed or central venous oxygen saturation; rSO_2: regional oxygen saturation; BUN: blood urea nitrogen; EF: ejection fraction; SF: shortening fraction; VTI: velocity time integral method)

- Loss of atrial contraction (may decrease CO by 25–30% in the presence of poor LV function).
- Acidosis:
  - Metabolic—tissue hypoperfusion.
  - Respiratory—hypoventilation.
- Electrolyte disturbances—low ionized calcium.
- Cardiac tamponade.

▌LOW CARDIAC OUTPUT

The assessment of low cardiac output states in infants and children requires the integration of clinical and monitoring techniques. In general, children compensate well for a low cardiac output by peripheral vasoconstriction and tachycardia such that a fall in arterial blood pressure is a late sign of cardiac decompression (Flowchart 3.1).

- Diagnosis:
  - Suspicion of low cardiac output is raised by evidence of peripheral vasoconstriction (cool, pale extremities, mottling, absent pedal pulses and capillary refill exceeding 3s), oliguria, metabolic acidosis and hyperthermia.
  - Increased lactate level on arterial blood gas.
  - Temperature gradient of more than 4–5° between the peripheral and core (rectum) temperature.
  - A narrow arterial pulse pressure, elevated filling pressures, low RA oxygen saturations and the development of atrial or ventricular arrhythmias also draw attention to a low cardiac output state.
- Treatment:
  - The treatment of a low cardiac output syndrome requires the assessment and manipulation of heart rate and rhythm, volume status, contractility and

Flowchart 3.1: Determinants of cardiac output and oxygen.

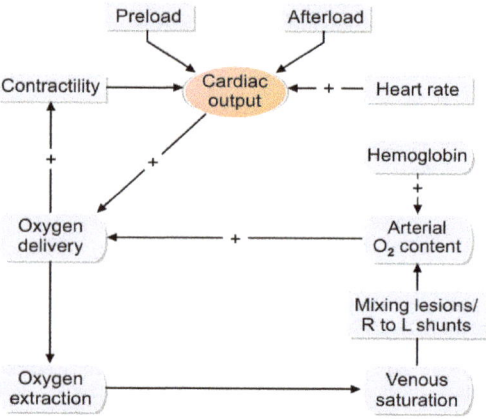

afterload. Each of these factors is discussed in the subsequent sections.

Additional contributory factors to a low cardiac output should be identified and treated. These may include:
- Cardiac tamponade (assessed by echocardiography).
- Ventilatory problems (chest X-ray to rule out severe pulmonary vascular congestion, atelectasis, pneumothorax, or large hemothorax; ABG's to identify hypoxia or hypercarbia).
- Metabolic problems (acidosis, hypo- or hyperkalemia, hypocalcemia).

HEART RATE AND RHYTHM

- If possible, the heart rate and rhythm should be optimized to achieve a regular supraventricular rhythm. The optimal heart rate is determined by the child's age (Table 3.2); the actual pulse rate will usually exceed the resting baseline values because of increased levels of circulating catecholamines and the use of inotropic drugs following surgery. Tachycardia is the most significant compensatory mechanism in children to maintain cardiac output, and may simply reflect hypovolemia that should be treated simultaneously.
- Sinus and nodal bradycardia should be treated with atrial pacing.
- Complete heart block, which may occur after operations requiring suturing near the AV node (VSD, AV canal), should be treated with AV sequential pacing. It is important to take advantage of the atrial contribution to filling in the early postoperative period.

TABLE 3.2: Average heart rates in children.

Age	Average heart rate	
	Mean	Range
Newborn	123	94–154
1–2 days	123	91–159
3–6 days	129	91–166
1–3 weeks	148	107–182
1–2 months	149	121–179
3–5 months	141	106–186
6–11 months	134	109–169
1–2 years	119	89–151
3–4 years	108	73–137
5–7 years	100	65–130
8–11 years	91	62–130
12–15 years	85	60–119

- Supraventricular tachyarrhythmias are more difficult to treat, but usually respond to digoxin, type IA antiarrhythmics, or electrical cardioversion, if necessary.
- Junctional ectopic tachycardia (JET), a potentially fatal arrhythmia, should treat aggressively (*see* Chapter 9: Cardiac Arrhythmias).

ACCEPTABLE PARAMETERS

Because each child's postoperative cardiac status is unique, initial acceptable parameters for blood pressure, RA and LA pressures, and urine output should be defined by the surgeon or cardiac anesthesiologist for the house staff and nurses at the time the patient arrives in the ICU. In the postoperative patient, there is a variation from normal baseline values for the resting child. Furthermore, there is frequently a change in myocardial performance and peripheral vasomotor tone during the early postoperative period that will require a redefinition of acceptable parameters.

- Systolic blood pressures for children of various ages are listed in Table 3.3.
- The usual range of postoperative RA and LA pressure is 8–12 mm Hg.

However, higher pressures are commonly required to optimize cardiac performance and depend on the specific cardiac lesion and the operative procedure.

- Urine output should exceed 1 mL/kg/h.
- *Special studies:* When cardiac performance following corrective surgery is not as expected and does not respond to standard therapeutic measures, early reinvestigation is recommended:
  - Unsuspected pericardial tamponade, ventricular dysfunction, inadequate or disrupted intracardiac repairs, or malfunctioning, prosthetic heart valves may be detected by echocardiography.
  - The intracardiac lines placed during surgery can be used to provide information on pressures, gradients and shunts.

TABLE 3.3: Normal blood pressure for various ages.

Ages	Mean systolic ± 2 SD	Mean diastolic ± 2 SD
Newborn	80 ± 16	46 ± 16
6 months–1 year	90 ± 25	50 ± 20
1–4 years	95 ± 25	65 ± 25
4–5 years	100 ± 20	65 ± 15
6–10 years	105 ± 15	57 ± 8
10–16 years	115 ± 19	60 ± 8

- The ratio of pulmonary blood flow to systemic blood flow (Qp/Qs) is calculated using the following formula:

$$(Qp/Qs) = \frac{\text{Aortic } O_2 \text{ sat} - \text{RA } O_2 \text{ sat}}{\text{LA } O_2 \text{ sat} - \text{PA } O_2 \text{ sat}}$$

- A shunt exceeding 2:1 usually requires reoperation, whereas one that is less than 1.5:1 is not hemodynamically significant. Shunts between 1.5:1 and 2:1 require further delineation of cardiac abnormalities and a careful assessment of the patient's clinical status.
- Cardiac catheterization may be required to define residual intracardiac lesions, such as a left-to-right shunt, and early diagnosis of treatable intracardiac pathology will allow reoperation before irreversible cardiac, pulmonary, renal neurologic and/or metabolic damage has developed.

VOLUME STATUS

- The optimal preload conditions for an individual patient depend on the specific congenital defect, the nature and adequacy of the repair, and the severity of right or left ventricular dysfunction. It is important to document the filling pressures (RA and LA pressures) both at the time of weaning from cardiopulmonary bypass (CPB) and on arrival in the ICU:
  - It is common to find that higher filling pressures are required 3–6 hours postoperatively, which corresponds to the time of maximal myocardial edema and dysfunction.
  - An acute change in filling pressures may result from a change in cardiac rhythm.
  - In neonates and infants, the anterior fontanelle can be assessed for volume status.
- When there is evidence of a low cardiac output syndrome, the volume status should be addressed while potential contributing causes are being evaluated. With hypovolemia, the LA pressure will be low (<10 mm Hg) and the arterial pressure tracing will display a narrow waveform reflective of a diminished stroke volume:
  - In addition, the normal respiratory variation in blood pressure noted during positive pressure ventilation will be exaggerated on the arterial display monitor.
  - Careful assessment of the input and output, with particular attention to urine output and chest tube drainage, is also helpful in assessing the degree of hypovolemia.
- In the absence of an LA line, a low CVP is consistent with hypovolemia. However, a high CVP may indicate right

ventricle (RV) dysfunction and/or elevated PVR. In either situation, volume infusion to normalize or increase the CVP may be required to ensure adequate left-sided filling.
- Hypovolemia should be treated with fluid replacement to expand the intravascular volume. Most centers use either blood or colloid (fresh frozen plasma or 5% albumin) as fluid boluses to maintain adequate preload. The selection of the particular fluid depends on the patient's hematocrit, clotting status and interval since surgery. Fluids are given in 5–10 mL/kg increments (6 to 12% of blood volume). Further volume infusion should be based on the hemodynamic response to each fluid bolus. An adequate response should be a rise in filling pressure and blood pressure with a decrease in heart rate and improvement in peripheral perfusion.

CARDIAC CONTRACTILITY AND AFTERLOAD

When systemic arterial hypotension or signs of low cardiac output persist after restoration of blood volume, then cardiac contractility and/or afterload require manipulation. These two factors must be considered together because of their intrinsic relationship and because most of the relevant pharmacologic agents affect both simultaneously. Almost all patients undergoing open-heart surgery for congenital heart disease will require some form of inotropic therapy to be weaned from CPB, and these medications are usually continued during the early postoperative period.

LEFT VENTRICLE AND SYSTEMIC VASCULAR RESISTANCE

- If a cardiac output persists after the LA pressure has been raised to 12–15 mm Hg by volume infusion, cardiac contractility is most likely impaired. Further volume infusion to an LA pressure of 15–18 mm Hg may be necessary to obtain more LV output by the starling mechanism.
- If high filling pressures are required, an inotropic drug with predominant β_1 activity should be administered. If the SVR is high, vasodilating agents are administered and the doses for pediatric patients are noted (*see* Appendix 1).
  - Dopamine increases contractility and heart rate and can be used up to 20 μg/kg/min without compromising renal perfusion.
  - Dobutamine improves contractility and increases heart rate, with less vasoconstrictive effects than dopamine.
  - When profound LV failure is present, milrinone is very helpful. Its combined inotrope and vasodilating

properties enhance both RV and LV output. They are therefore beneficial in patients with either AV valve regurgitation or pulmonary hypertension.
- Epinephrine in low doses (0.01–0.1 µg/kg/min) is a strong inotrope and chronotrope that is commonly used in neonates undergoing complicated cardiac repairs.

(For dose and infusion, kindly *see* Appendix 1).
- Contractility refers to the intrinsic strength of myocardial contraction. In congenital heart disease, it is more common to see impairment of RV function, primarily because of preexisting pulmonary hypertension of volume overload.
- Afterload refers to ventricular wall tension during systole:
  - LV function may be improved by a reduction in LA pressure and SVR. This is beneficial in patients with systemic hypertension or residual AV valve regurgitation.
  - RV function may be improved by a reduction in RV volume and PVR. This is particularly important in neonates and young infants in whom reduction in PVR is essential to maintain RV performance:
    - Isoproterenol produces primarily an increase in heart rate, but also improves contractility and reduces PVR. Therefore, it is most beneficial for children with RV dysfunction. The tachycardia is well tolerated and often beneficial in small children.
    - For cardiac failure unresponsive to drug management, intra-aortic balloon counter pulsation can be considered in the older pediatric patient.
    - For large children or adolescents, an LV assist device may be used. Extracorporeal membrane oxygenation (ECMO) can be used for cardiopulmonary failure after bypass.

RIGHT VENTRICLE AND PULMONARY HYPERTENSION

- One of the significant differences between adult and pediatric cardiac surgical patients is the common occurrence of reactive pulmonary hypertension in children, which may predispose them to episodes of oxygen desaturation and RV failure:
  - Elevated PVR, whether fixed or dynamic, is often noted in patients with large left-to-right shunts and increased pulmonary blood flow. Coexisting high PVR and an impaired RV is a very dangerous combination. The contribution of an elevated PVR to RV failure is difficult to ascertain unless PA pressures and

cardiac outputs can be determined. Nonetheless, the treatment of RV dysfunction usually includes efforts to dilate the pulmonary vascular bed.
- The RV may also be predisposed to postoperative failure as a consequence of:
  - Underdevelopment.
  - Chronic high-pressure loading (hypertrophy).
  - Less-effective intraoperative myocardial protection.
  - Right ventriculotomy incisions.
  - Interruption of right coronary artery branches.
  - Residual pulmonary stenosis or insufficiency or tricuspid insufficiency.
- The assessment of RV function depends on clinical signs as well as a comparison of RA and LA pressure measurements. Clinically signs of RV failure include:
  - Jugular venous distension.
  - Hepatomegaly.
  - Peripheral edema.
  - Ascites.
  - Periorbital, flank and eventually generalized edema.
  - Rising blood urea nitrogen (BUN).

An elevated RA pressure with low LA pressure confirms the diagnosis of RV dysfunction. Volume loading to improve cardiac output will raise the RA pressure with proportionately less effect on the LA pressure.

- Treatment of RV failure:
  - Volume loading, often to an RA pressure of 15 mm Hg or greater, may be necessary to ensure adequate left-sided filling.
  - Use of an inotropic agent that may also produce pulmonary vasodilation should be selected. These include the following:
    - Low-dose dopamine/dobutamine.
    - Milrinone.
    - Sequential pacing if not in sinus rhythm.
    - Right ventricular assist device for older children.

Chapter 4

Respiratory Assessment and Management

M Gokulakrishnan

RESPIRATORY MANAGEMENT

- Children undergoing uncomplicated repairs—such as PDA ligation, coarctation repair or closure of and ASD—may be extubated in the operating room or soon after arrival in the ICU. They should be given supplemental oxygen and observed carefully for signs of respiratory distress. These include tachypnea, tachycardia, intercostal retraction, nasal flaring, grunting and gasping. Spontaneous respiratory rates will vary according to the age (Table 4.1).
- Patients undergoing more complex repair will require mechanical ventilation for a longer period after returning to ICU.

ENDOTRACHEAL (ET) TUBES

- Both cuffed and uncuffed endotracheal tubes are acceptable for intubation in infants and children. However, the trend is moving towards using cuffed tubes for all ages.
- In the operating room, cuffed endotracheal tubes are associated with a higher likelihood of correct selection of tube size, thus achieving a lower reintubation rate with no increased risk of perioperative complications.

TABLE 4.1: Normal respiratory rates in children.

Age	Respiratory rate
Newborn	40–6
1 month–1 year	30
2–4 years	26
4–6 years	22
6–8 years	21
8–10 years	20
10–12 years	19
12–14 years	18

- Cuff inflating pressure should be monitored and limited according to manufacturer's instruction (usually less than 20 to 25 cm H_2O).
- With the use of any uncuffed tube, a leak of more than 10 cm H_2O and less than 35 cm H_2O should be present during mechanical ventilation.
- Orotracheal route is the preferred option over nasotracheal route. Nasotracheal intubation has risks of nasal damage, sinusitis and local abscesses and its use is limited.
- Because of the necessity of longer and narrower tubes for the nasal route, pulmonary toileting is more difficult and airway resistance is greater.

Selection of Endotracheal Tube Size
- Infant-cuffed: 3.0 mm ID; Uncuffed: 3.5 mm ID.
  For 1 to 12 years of age use the following guideline formula:
- Cuffed ET tube: (Age/4) + 4 mm ID.
- Uncuffed ET tube: (Age/4) + 4 mm ID.
- Note that the size for cuffed is one size smaller than uncuffed tube.

ET tube fixation length =
  (Age/2) + 12 cm for oral tube
  (Age/2) + 15 cm for nasal tube.

MECHANICAL VENTILATORS
- **Pressure-limited ventilators** provide an inspiratory volume that is determined by a preset peak airway pressure. They are commonly used for neonates and infants less than 1 year of age who are more susceptible to barotrauma (pneumothorax or pneumomediastinum). This technique may deliver a variable amount of volume and give no assessment of change in lung compliance.
- **Volume-limited ventilators** deliver a present tidal volume usually at constant flow rates. A peak pressure limit alarm is utilized to prevent the development of excessive pressures, which could lead to barotrauma. Alarming may draw attention to changes in ventilatory mechanics (system malfunction, pneumothorax). These ventilators are preferred in older children in whom higher airway pressures are better tolerated and maintenance of a constant tidal volume helps to prevent atelectasis. They can be used as pressure-limited ventilators in younger children by setting a peak pressure to limit the tidal volume.
- **Time-cycled ventilators** deliver a tidal volume determined by both inspiratory time and flow rate. At intermittent intervals, the gas flow is interrupted by a

time-cycled expiratory valve. A prolonged inspiratory phase can increase mean airway pressure (similar to a volume-limited system) and improve oxygenation, but it may reduce gas escape during a shorter expiratory phase. These ventilators offer more control over the respiratory cycle, helping the clinician adjust mechanical ventilation to the specific needs of the patient. They are commonly used in infants.
- Regardless of which type of ventilator is used, vigilant attention to the oxygen flow rates delivered by the ventilator, expiratory volumes, auscultation of bilateral breath sounds, chest wall expansion, arterial blood gas (ABG) analysis and hemodynamic parameters is essential. Changes in ventilator settings should be based on these assessments.

VENTILATOR SETTING

Preferred Modes

Neonates—pressure control ventilation (PCV):
- 6-8 kg—preferably PCV.
- 8-10 kg—synchronized intermittent mandatory ventilation (SIMV)/volume control (VC).

Setting up a Volume-Controlled Ventilation

- *Set tidal volume:* 10-12 mL/kg.
- Respiratory rate according to the age (*see* Table 4.1).
- Set FiO_2 (initially set at 1.0, reduce as indicated).
- Set alarms for MV, peak pressures, positive end-expiratory pressure (PEEP).
- *Set inspiratory time*—usually at 25% of respiratory cycle: 1:2 (normal). It can be 1:1 or even 2:1 in case of acute respiratory distress syndrome (ARDS).
- *Set PEEP:* Usually 3-5 cm H_2O.

Pressure Control Ventilator

- Set inspiratory pressure between 15 and 20 cm H_2O, judged by degree of chest expansion.
- Set frequency—choose mode of ventilation (triggered or mandatory).
- Set inspiratory time to 0.6 to 1.0s, depending on age.
- Set alarms.
- Set FiO_2.
- *Set PEEP:* 3-5 cm H_2O.

Setting up Synchronized Intermittent Mandatory Ventilation

Volume-controlled SIMV

Set TV: 8-10 mL/kg:
- Set RR according to age and $ETCO_2$.

- Set PEEP (usually 3–5 cm H_2O).
- Set trigger—usually 0.5 to 1 in neonates/small children.
- Set inspiratory time to get I:E ratio of 1:2.
- Peak pressure support is usually 10 cm H_2O.
- Peak flow (children: 20 l/min, adult: 30 l/min).
- FiO_2: To maintain PO_2 of 100 mm Hg.

Setting up Pressure-Controlled SIMV
- Set PC to achieve expiratory tidal volume of 8–10 mL/kg.
- Rest same as VSIMV.

High-Frequency Oscillation Ventilation
Consult with the Intensivist if high-frequency oscillation ventilation (HFOV) is considered.

MANAGEMENT OF CHILDREN DURING MECHANICAL VENTILATION

- All children require sedation during mechanical ventilation. This prevents inadvertent dislodgment of the endotracheal tube, improves the efficiency of gas exchange and minimizes the development of paroxysmal pulmonary hypertension and arterial desaturation.
- Opioids and muscle relaxants used during surgery are not reversed, and the child requires additional medications for pain and agitation. Continuous infusions are commonly used in children because they can maintain a more constant level of analgesia with use of less medication. Medications may include the following:
  – Analgesics and sedatives:
    - Morphine, 0.05–0.1 mg/kg q1–2 h or 10–40 µg/kg/h continuous infusions.
    - Fentany, 2–5 µg/kg/h continuous infusion; tolerance to this short-acting narcotic may develop, necessitating increasing doses to maintain the same level of analgesia.
    - Midazolam, 0.05–0.2 mg/kg, then 0.4–1.2 µg/kg/min infusion; this may have a synergistic depressant effect on myocardial function when used with fentanyl.
  – Muscle relaxants:
    - Vecuronium, 0.1 mg/kg, then 0.05–0.1 mg/kg/h infusion.
    - Pancuronium, 0.1 mg/kg, then 0.05–0.1 mg/kg/h infusion (this increases sympathetic tone and may increase the heart rate).
- Oxygenation criteria differ depending on the nature of the congenital heart defect and the surgical procedure. Following total anatomic or physiologic correction, a PO_2 >80 torr with an FiO_2 of 0.4 should be expected. However,

following palliative procedures for cyanotic defects with continued shunting or intracardiac mixing, an oxygen saturation of 75–85% (PaO_2 of 40–50 torr) is anticipated. In the presence of severe V/Q mismatch or a residual shunt, use of 100% oxygen is incapable of improving oxygenation significantly. The addition of positive end-expiratory pressure (PEEP) (5 cm H_2O) to the ventilatory circuitry may be of some benefit in maintaining functional residual capacity and minimizing atelectasis, especially in children with large left-to-right shunts. PEEP should be avoided after a Fontan operation, Glenn procedure.

- The FiO_2 is gradually lowered to 0.4 if oxygenation remains satisfactory. This can be assessed continuously by pulse oximetry and confirmed by intermittent ABG analysis.
- Several physiologic factors unique to the pediatric patient population should be taken into consideration:
  - The pulmonary vasculature is sensitive to changes in PO_2 and PCO_2; hypoxia or hypercarbia may produce paroxysmal pulmonary hypertension, which can lead to arterial desaturation and right ventricular decompensation.
  - As the endotracheal tubes are so small in children, heated humidification of inspired gases is essential to prevent the drying of secretions and the airway mucosa.
  - Infants depend primarily on the diaphragm to perform the work of breathing. Any impairment of diaphragmatic function (paresis, abdominal distention) can lead to respiratory compromise. This can be assessed by an X-ray (diaphragm will be higher than normal) or by a bedside 2D echo when the child is spontaneously breathing.

WEANING AND EXTUBATION

- Several days of intubation are beneficial for children with large left-to-right shunts, significant pulmonary hypertension (ratio of PA/systemic pressure greater than 0.75) and young infants undergoing complex cardiac repairs. Weaning is generally accomplished using the intermittent mandatory ventilation (IMV) mode:
  - In infants, the IMV rate is lowered by 2–4 breaths/min and PEEP is decreased to 2–3 cm H_2O. Weaning to continuous positive airway pressure (CPAP) without any positive pressure breaths should be avoided because the endotracheal tube increases airway resistance, the work of breathing and diaphragmatic fatigue.

- In older children, the IMV rate is lowered by 2-4 breaths/min to CPAP. PEEP is gradually reduced in 2-3 cm increments to 3-5 cm H_2O.
  - If the duration of intubation is short, extubation can usually be accomplished from 4 breaths/min if the criteria listed below are met.
- Criteria for weaning and extubation include:
  - Adequate level of consciousness.
  - Hemodynamic stability with minimal mediastinal bleeding (<1 mL/kg/h) and adequate peripheral perfusion.
  - Normothermia.
  - PaO_2 > 8 torr on FiO_2 < 0.4 (40 torr, if residual right-to-lift shunting).
  - pH: 7.35-7.45.
  - Vital capacity >10-15 mL/kg (crying VC >15 mL/kg in infants).
  - Maximum negative force against an occluded airway > 20-30 cm H_2O (>45 cm H_2O infants).
- Humidified oxygen should be given by mask after extubation with rechecking of an ABG within 30 minutes. Subsequently, chest physiotherapy is used to stimulate coughing and mobilize secretions.
- Children may develop airway obstruction from subglottic edema following extubation. This is usually treated with nebulized racemic epinephrine (0.5 mL/kg diluted to 2 mL of normal saline q2h to maximum dose of 0.5 mL). If duration of intubation has been prolonged or there is minimal leak around an uncuffed tube, suggesting the presence of significant subglottic edema, then use of dexamethasone 0.2-0.5 mg/kg IV q4-qh for two doses before extubation may be beneficial.
- The child should be prevented from struggling on ventilator on CPAP mode.

Chapter 5

Pulmonary Hypertension Crisis and Management

Prashant Shah

PULMONARY HYPERTENSIVE CRISIS
Definition of Pulmonary Hypertension
A paroxysmal increase in pulmonary artery pressure to systemic or suprasystemic levels, associated with a low cardiac output and a low left atrial pressure. This is generally preceded by a progressive but rapid increase in pulmonary artery pressure without a decrease in systemic pressure. This sign should be carefully sought and action should start at this point without waiting for a PHC to be established. If unrecognized or not treated properly, it can be fatal. This is a special situation that may occur in patients who have had high-flow left-to-right shunts or obstructed pulmonary venous return with increased pulmonary vascular reactivity, e.g. VSD, AVSD, TAPVD, TGA + VSD, truncus arteriosus, AP window.

Diagnosis of PHC
- Increase pulmonary artery pressure.
- Increase right atrium (RA) pressure.
- Desaturation.
- Bradycardia.
- Lower arterial blood pressure.

Precipitating Factors
- Residual shunt or stenosis.
- Fall in arterial PO_2.
- Fall in pH.
- Acidosis.
- Stimulation—ET suction, chest physio, inadequate sedation.
- Sepsis, respiratory infection.

Preventive Measures
- Start Inj Milrinone or Inj Phenoxybenzamine to lower PA pressure.
- Ventilate patient adeguetely and keep PaO_2 > 100 mm Hg and PCO_2 30–35 mm Hg.

- To maintain pH at a level that restricts a rise in PVR ($PaCO_2$: 35 mm Hg; pH >7.40).
- Deep sedation—fentanyl at 5–10 μg/kg/h—with adequate loading dose and boluses prior to stimulating procedures.
- Avoid positive end-expiratory pressure (PEEP) >4.
- Start tablet sildenafil 1–2 mg/kg/day in 3–4 divided doses via NG tube; give first dose in OT after induction.
- Establish FiO_2 of 1.0 on return from theater; gradually reduce FiO_2 according to blood gases to maintain an arterial PO_2 >100 mm Hg.
- Consider inhaled nitric oxide early if PAP does not come down with other measures as described earlier.
- Phenoxybenzamine may already have been given in the operating room; continue at a dose of 1 mg/kg 12 hourly.
- Endotracheal suction only if required and precede it by a bolus of sedation and preoxygenation by hand-bagging. If physiotherapy induces PHC, then review the management with the consultant.
- Rule out any residual lesion.

Therapeutic Measures
- Hand-bagging with 100% oxygen.
- Increase sedation and paralyze the child.
- Consider inhaled nitric oxide.
- Tablet sildenafil or bosentan through Ryle's tube (consider tablet bosentan only after baseline normal liver function).
- Inj Sildenafil (10 mg/12.5 mL) is available start with 0.3 mg/kg Bolus over 30 minutes followed by 1.6 mg/kg/d infusion for 48 hours.
- Injection phenoxybenzamine and/or injection milrinone.
- 'Nitric oxide (NO)' is an agent of choice. It should be used only if other measures are ineffective.
- When inhaled with oxygen, it induces relaxation of pulmonary vascular smooth muscle. It has few systemic side effects, as it avidly binds to Hb in circulation and inactivates it.
- Dose is 10–80 ppm and must be closely regulated as higher concentration can be toxic to the lungs. Test dose should be of 50 ppm.

Weaning
If the child is stable for 24 hours, the order in which the child is weaned from its support is as follows:
- Gradually allow pH to fall to 7.40.
- Stop paralysis.
- Wean FiO_2 to 0.6.
- Wean nitric oxide.
- Reduce sedation.
- Stop phenoxybenzamine only after extubation.
- Continue tablet sildenafil and/or bosentan for 3 months.

Chapter 6

Fluid and Electrolyte Management

G Selvakumar, Shrishu Kamath, Karthik Surya

INTRODUCTION

- Patients who return to the ICU following surgery with cardiopulmonary bypass (CPB) typically have significant total body water and salt overload from dilution of blood with crystalloid in the bypass circuit (e.g. to a hematocrit of 20%).
- Neonates and young infants appear to acquire a relatively greater excess of fluid than older children, at times experiencing intraoperative weight gains of 600–1000 g (20–25% of preoperative weight). The additional fluid distributes diffusely throughout the body, including into the soft tissues, lungs, kidneys, brain and myocardium. The mechanism for this process appears to be a generalized capillary leak from endothelial damage caused by exposure to CPB and/or ischemia-reperfusion injury.
- In anticipation of this extracellular fluid overload, some institutions employ strategies such as ultrafiltration during the final period of CPB or routine placement of a peritoneal dialysis.
- In the first 2–4 hours following admission to the ICU, most patients who have undergone CPB produce more than 1 mL/kg/h of urine. The brief initial period of increased output occurs by an osmotic diuresis. This osmotic diuresis is caused either by the elevated glucose level of the CPB priming solution causing hyperglycemia and the stress response to surgery or intraoperative mannitol administration. During the 12–18 hours after the hyperglycemia and glycosuria resolve, the kidneys often respond poorly to diuretic agents, in part because of the inappropriate secretion of antidiuretic hormone (SIADH). Therefore, diuretic therapy is typically initiated on postoperative day 1, because it is seldom effective before that time.
- In the first 24 hours, the total rate of intravenous (IV) fluid administration is typically set at one-half to two-thirds

of the maintenance fluid rate. The maintenance fluid rate can be calculated using the surface area method (maintenance = 1500–1700 mL/m^2/d).

Day of operation	1 mL/kg/h = 24 mL/kg/day
1st postoperative day	2 mL/kg/h = 48 mL/kg/day
2nd postoperative day	3 mL/kg/h = 72 mL/kg/day
3rd postoperative day	4 mL/kg/h = 96 mL/kg/day

OR

Open heart surgery:
1000 mL/m^2/day on day of surgery
       (BSA = Height × Weight/3600)
1st day of surgery = 1250 mL/m^2/day
Closed heart surgery:
<10 kg = 80–100 mL/kg/day
10 kg = 80–100% of normal fluid requirement
Normal fluid requirement:
1–10 kg = 100 mL/kg/day
11–20 kg = 1000 mL + mL/kg/day
21–40 kg = 1500 mL + 20 mL/kg/day
For example, for a 15 kg child: 1–10 kg = 100 mL/kg is 1000 mL + 5 kg = 50 mL/kg is 250 mL, so normal requirement will be 1250 mL/day.

Patients who undergo CPB should be fluid-restricted for at least the first 72 hours postoperatively. The following levels of fluid restriction are used:

These fluid restriction levels and further increments in volume depend on the clinical condition of the patient and should be checked with the consultant-in-charge of the ward round.

- Examples of situations in which a maintenance or greater IV fluid rate is appropriate would be the following:
  - Modified Blalock-Taussig shunt in the polycythemic patient to decrease the risks of both inadequate shunt flow from low intravascular volume and shunt thrombosis.
  - Cavopulmonary anastomosis or Fontan procedure to provide adequate preload for nonpulsatile pulmonary blood flow.
  - The patient with normal blood pressure after aortic coarctation repair, a procedure performed without CPB and typically not accompanied by fluid overload.

- A thorough assessment of the postoperative patient's fluid balance and electrolytes status should be made at least once a day in the ICU. Sources of data for this assessment include physical examination, monitored variables such as systemic blood pressure, central venous pressure (CVP) or right atrial pressure (Rap), LA (if available), heart rate, and fluid input and output volumes, and laboratory determinations of serum electrolytes, blood urea nitrogen, creatinine, hematocrit and urinalysis.
- Daily weight measurement can be useful.
- The type of fluid to infuse depends on the knowledge of the patient's postoperative physiology, hematocrit, coagulation status and type of ongoing fluid losses.

TYPES OF FLUIDS

- Newborn <2 days—10% dextrose:
  - >2 days and infants—1/2 DNS (10 or 5%) or isolyte P.
  - >1 years—1/2 DNS (5%) or isolyte P.
- Fluids changed according to blood sugars, serum Na, serum K levels.
- Colloidal solution—20% albumin (1 mL/kg/h for 5 hours):
  - Dextran, fresh frozen plasma (FFP) can also be used as volume expanders.
  - 5% Albumin can be used as boluses for maintaining CVP.
- Blood glucose and serum electrolyte measurements should be made within 1 hour of admission to the ICU every 4-6 hours during the initial 24 hours after surgery in higher-risk patients.
- Potassium, primarily in the form of potassium chloride (KCl), is added to the IV fluid solution to treat low serum K^+.

Potassium chloride may need to be prescribed in postbypass patients to correct hypokalemia or ameliorate potassium losses from diuretic therapy and/or high urinary output (*Note:* most postbypass patients receive a stat dose of frusemide in the theater) (*see* sections on hypokalemia and hyperkalemia for further details). Arterial. CVP, pulmonary artery pressure (PAP), left atrial pressure (LAP) flushing is normally 0.9% NaCl at 0.5-1 mL/h. For patients <1 year of age, 10% dextrose is used to prepare infusion drugs. 10% dextrose should not be used for LA line. If plasma sodium is low, 10 or 5% dextrose/0.45% NaCl may be substituted as maintenance solution.

BLOOD REPLACEMENT

- Blood losses should be replaced with:
  - Packed cells (or whole blood).
  - FFP according to the Hb.
- All blood should be crossmatched—if not previously crossmatched.
- All blood products (apart from PPF) need to be obtained from the transfusion department.
- The laboratory has to be contacted by phone to obtain FFP/platelets/cryoprecipitate.
- FFP and platelets should be group specific (transfusion incompatibility has been seen with both).
- The Hb desired is 12 g/dL for noncyanotic patients and 14 g/dL for cyanotic patients.

HYPERKALEMIA

Causes: Low cardiac output, hemolysis, renal failure (prerenal and renal), over dosage, acidosis:

- Check blood for hemolysis and acid-base balance, and confirm the value of pH.
- Both the absolute value and the rate of rise of K are important, but do not ignore a single high K value.
- Check urine output.
- Check cardiac output and improve if necessary.
- Remove K from IV fluids and any oral supplements; stop K-sparing drugs:
  - If K >5 and urine output <2 mL/kg/h give frusemide 1 mg/kg.
  - Consider lowering the serum potassium by:
    - Increasing alkalosis (respiratory or metabolic) Full correction = Weight × Base excess deficit × 0.3.
    - Insulin and glucose (0.1 u/kg insulin with 2 mL/kg 50% dextrose).

    OR
    - 10 mL of D25 with 1 mL of plain insulin (1 mL = 4 unit of insulin).
    - Dose 0.1 iu/kg as a bolus or infusion.
    - Injection 10% calcium gluconate: 1–2 mg/kg IV slowly.
- Salbutamol bolus (5 µg/kg) and infusion at up to 5 µg/kg/h or nebulization.
- Calcium resonium (250–500 mg/kg PR or oral for 6 hours diluted with 20% sorbitol or 25% dextrose):
  - or sodium polystyrene sulfonate (Kayexalate): 0.3–0.6 mg/kg/dose PO/PR for 6 hours:
    - Dialysis—peritoneal.
    - Hemodialysis.

- If there are changes in the ECG (Fig. 6.1) consistent with hyperkalemia, consider IV calcium (0.5 mL/kg 10% calcium gluconate) as an infusion.
- These are all temporary measures, and if the underlying cause is not improved or eliminated then consider the need to institute acute renal support.

HYPOKALEMIA

Following CPB, levels below 3.5 mEq/L may be associated with cardiac dysrhythmias.

Serum K^+ <3.5 mmol/L

Add 10 mmol KCl to 100 mL b of infusion fluid in a burette and deliver at standard rate for maintenance fluid.

For children

Injection KCl—0.3 mEq/kg diluted in 20 mL fluid infused over 20 minutes time.

If the amount of KCl is more than 10 mEq then dilute in 50 mL fluid and infuse over 20 minutes.

Oral—Syrup KCl

- Less than 5 years—1 mEq/kg/dose (15 mL = 20 mEq).
- More than 5 kg—0.5 mEq/kg/dose:
  - Do not flush bolus.

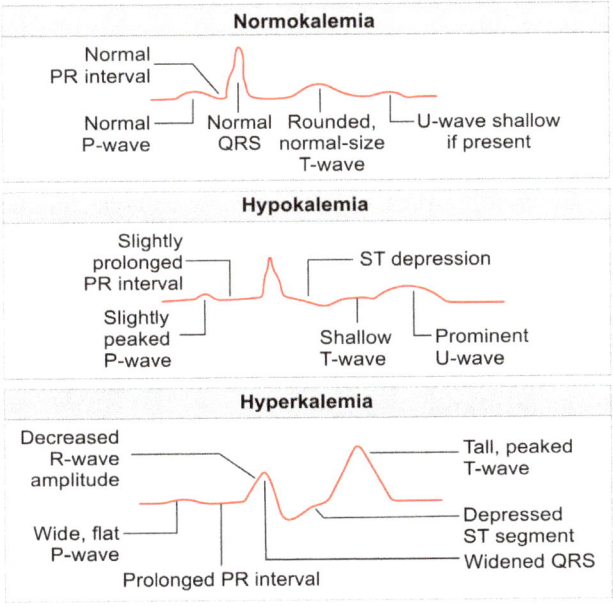

Fig. 6.1: ECG changes and serum potassium (K^+).

- Keep syringe separately.
- Check K⁺ level for every 2 hours.

Serum K⁺ <2.5 mmol/L

Add 20 mmol to 40 mL normal saline and deliver at a maximum rate of 0.5 mL/kg/h via a syringe pump; this line must not be flushed. Check K⁺ at least for every 2 hours until normalization. Review diuretic therapy.

The use of strong potassium infusions needs careful consideration outside the immediate postoperative period and any patient on a strong potassium infusion needs careful and repeated serum potassium analysis. Strong potassium infusions should only be administered on central lines to prevent the associated problems of extravasation. Strong potassium infusions can be extremely dangerous and lead to cardiac arrest if appropriate monitoring is not carried out.

Following the immediate postoperative day, potassium supplementation needs to be individually assessed for each patient, and with sequential increases in fluid volume the above concentrations of potassium chloride may be in excess of that required to maintain serum potassium.

Diuretic therapy—usually instigated on day 1—can be accompanied by oral amiloride using 0.2 mg/kg per dose if the patient is tolerating NGT feeds.

Note: Patients on ACE inhibitors should not be prescribed amiloride, especially if they are about to return to the cardiac ward.

HYPERNATREMIA (FLOWCHART 6.1)

Serum Na⁺ >150 mEq/L

Causes

- Vomiting/diarrhea, excess water loss, osmotic diuretics, burns, diabetes insipidus (DI).
- High sodium intake.
- Near drowning.

Clinical Features

- Lethargy, irritability, coma, altered mental state, seizures.
- Complain of polyuria or thirst.
- Severity of symptoms related to rise in plasma Na⁺ concentration.
- Mortality 45% in acute hypernatremia.

Treatment

- Treat underlying cause.
- Correction = (serum Na – expected Na) × 0.6 × Weight.

- Expected Na OR water deficit = [Plasma (Na^+) concentration−140]/140 × total body water.
- IVF—1/2 DNS, slow correction of sodium (0.5–1 mEq/L/h).
- Rapid correction of hypernatremia is dangerous.
- Desmopressin in DI to reduce water loss.
- Do not use plain dextrose IVF to correct sodium as it can cause cerebral edema and seizures.

HYPONATREMIA (FLOWCHARTS 6.2 AND 6.3)

Serum Na^+ <115 mEq/L

Causes

- Inappropriate ADH secretion—decrease water clearance.
- Excess water—nephritic syndrome, heart failure, liver failure.
- Excess Na loss—diuretics, renal tubular dysfunction, vomit, diarrhea, burns, peritonitis.
- Hyperglycemia, hyperlipidemia, hyperproteinemia.

Clinical Features

Patient can present with varying degree of severity from asymptomatic to coma, nausea, vomiting, irritability, lethargy, delirium, drowsiness, seizures.

Treatment

- Fluid restriction.
- Slow correction of Na over 24–48 hours.

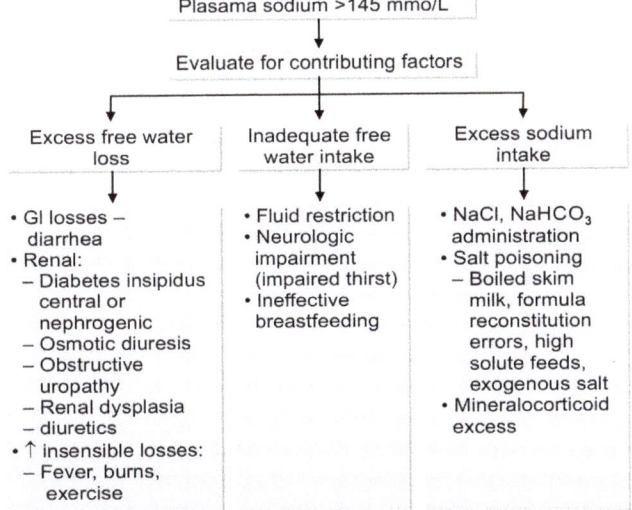

Flowchart 6.1: Diagnostic approach to hypernatremia.

Flowchart 6.2: Management of underlying causes of hyponatremia.

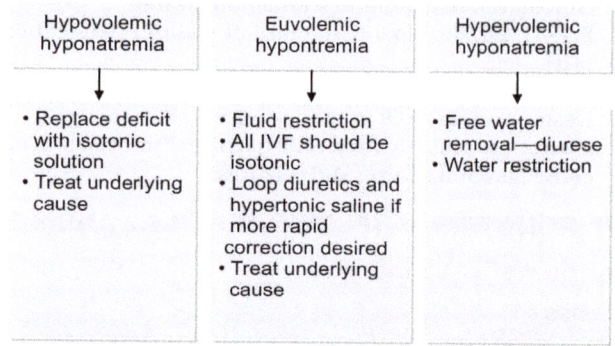

- 3% NaCl—1 mL/min (max: 12 mL/kg) only if patient is symptomatic (seizures).
- IVF—RL OR NS can be used along with K^+ supplementation.

Correction = (135−serum Na) × 0.6 × Wt. + daily req. of Na (3–4 mEq/kg/day).

MAGNESIUM DEFICIENCY

Low magnesium levels can cause cardiac arrhythmias, pulmonary hypertension, poor respiratory function, paresthesiae, fits, tetany and bronchoconstriction. It can exacerbate digoxin toxicity.

Common causes of magnesium depletion are diuretic therapy with accompanying hypokalemia, hypocalcemia, diarrhea, diabetic ketoacidosis and dietary deficit.

Supplementation

Low magnesium levels are usually supplemented by the IV route—oral magnesium is a potent laxative and will cause diarrhea. Patients on TPN can have their magnesium levels increased in the TPN solution.

Dose

- Use 50% magnesium sulfate (2 mmol/mL).
- Dilute 0.2 mL/kg (= 0.4 mmol/kg) in either 5% dextrose or 0.9% NaCl.
- Give as slow IV infusion over 30–60 minutes for every 12 hours.

HYPOCALCEMIA

Low calcium levels are often seen in postoperative cardiac patients. The biochemical analysis of the pathology department provides both a serum calcium level and a corrected (for albumin) calcium level. The physiologically

Fluid and Electrolyte Management

Flowchart 6.3: Diagnostic approach to hyponatremia.

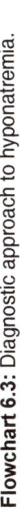

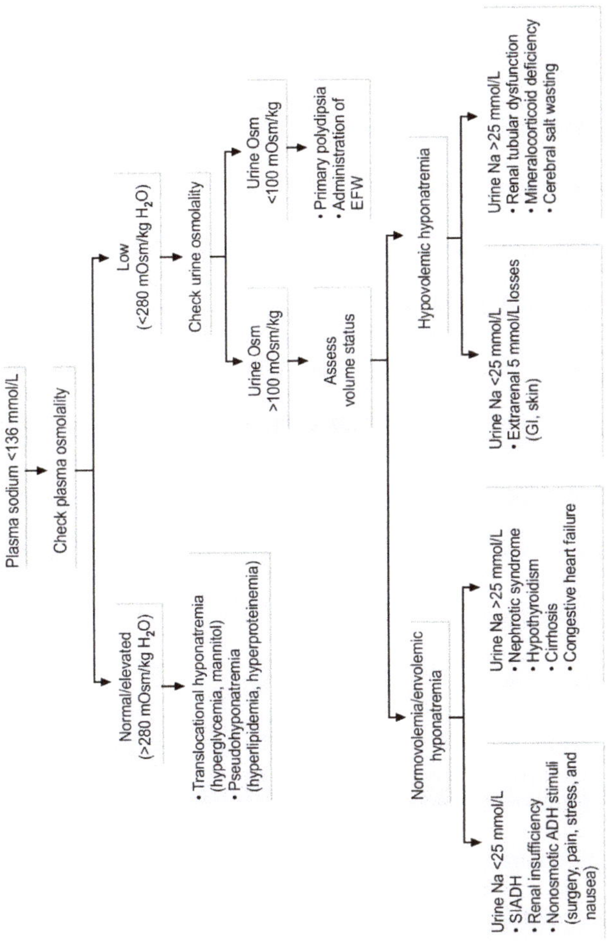

active component is the ionized calcium, which can be analyzed on both blood gas machines on the unit.

Common causes of hypocalcemia are:
- Excessive blood transfusion (citrate used in the preservation of stored blood binds to calcium).
- Renal failure.
- DiGeorge syndrome.

Hypocalcemia is associated with reduced ventricular function and cardiac arrhythmias, i.e. prolonged Q-T interval.

Supplementation

During large blood transfusion, often necessary when patients are bleeding postoperatively, 1 mL of 10% calcium gluconate can be given by slow IV infusion for every 100 mL of blood transfused:
- Hypocalcemia can be corrected by slow IV infusion of 0.5 mL/kg 10% calcium gluconate solution to a maximum of 20 mL.
- In cases of severe hypocalcemia a continuous IV infusion of 10% calcium gluconate can be given at the rate of 0.2 mL/kg/h.
- Injection calcium chloride 10% 0.2 mL/kg as bolus or injection calcium gluconate 10%–0.5–1 mL/kg as bolus.

PROTOCOL FOR METABOLIC ACIDOSIS

Indication

Metabolic acidosis exists if the base deficit is >2 mEq/L and pH is <7.35 or $PaCO_2$ is <30 mm Hg.

Rationale

Treatment is directed only at the extracellular fluid and only a conservative dose of $NaHCO_3$ is given, because more can easily be administered, if needed.

Look for underlying cause like low CO_2, hypovolemia, hypo- or hyperglycemia, hypothermia.

Extracellular fluid volume = 30% body weight (kg).
Base deficit (mEq/L) × 0.3 × Body weight (kg) = total extracellular base deficit.

TREATMENT

- Administer $NaHCO_3$, so that the amount of Na^+ (mEq) equals half the total extracellular base deficit.
- Remeasure the base deficit in 30–60 minutes and repeat treatment if indicated.

Note: In acute reduction of cardiac output or cardiac arrest, much larger doses of $NaHCO_3$ are indicated (44 mEq for adults, 1 mEq/kg for infants and children).

Chapter 7

Mediastinal Bleeding, Cardiac Tamponade and Transfusion Therapy

Amit Mishra

MEDIASTINAL BLEEDING AND TRANSFUSION THERAPY

- Mediastinal bleeding in the pediatric patient following open-heart surgery can lead to rapid hemodynamic deterioration and must be treated aggressively. Tamponade may occur with as little as 10–20 mL of blood within the mediastinum in the small child. Children at increased risk of mediastinal bleeding include those with the following:
  - Cyanotic conditions.
  - Impaired coagulation status (neonates).
  - Hepatic congestion from right ventricular (RV) failure.
  - Use of profound hypothermia with circulatory arrest during surgery.
  - Complicated reoperative procedure.
- Coagulation studies [prothrombin time (PT), partial thromboplastin time (PTT), platelet count] should be sent upon arrival in the ICU. The management of mediastinal bleeding should ideally be based on the results of these studies, but empiric therapy is usually required when there is significant bleeding and results are not available.
- The postoperative hematocrit should be maintained at 40–45% for patients with continued cyanosis (following palliative procedures with residual shunts or intracardiac mixing) and at 35–40% for all others. Ideally, fresh whole blood should be used, if available, because it contains platelets and clotting factors:
  - Transfusion of red cells should be based on the most recent hematocrit. If there is ongoing chest tube bleeding, packed red cells, frequently in combination with fresh frozen plasma, may be given in a total volume equal to the previous hour's losses.
  - Autotransfusion systems are available and are most useful when the child requires volumes and red cells, rather than a concentrated red cell transfusion (HCT of a unit of packed RBCs = 70%). Small additional

doses of protamine should be given when blood processed with a cell-saving device is administered.
- Cold blood should never be transfused; it should be allowed to warm before transfusion or should be administered through a warming device.
- The administration of blood products should always be tempered by the potential for transmission of infectious disease and the possibility of febrile, allergic or transfusion reactions.
- The amount of packed red cells to be given to achieve a specified hematocrit can be determined by the following equation:
Packed cells transfused (mL) = Est. blood volume × $(HCT_{desired} - HCT_{actual})/HCT_{packed\ cells}$
Or more simply:
Packed cells transfused (mL) = [70 × Wt (kg) × HCT]/70 = Wt (kg) × (HCT).
- Citrate toxicity from massive transfusion is very uncommon; however, if transfusions exceeding one-half of the patient's blood volume are administered (i.e. more than 35 mL/kg), 1 mL of calcium gluconate (10% solution) per 100 mL of transfused blood should be given through a peripheral line.
- The use of fractionated blood products should be based on the results of the coagulation studies. A prolonged PTT with normal PT suggests heparin excess; 0.5–1.0 mg/kg of protamine sulfate is given.
- A prolonged PT and PTT suggests depletion of coagulation factors; 10 mL/kg of fresh frozen plasma (FFP) is given. Cryoprecipitate is rich in factors I and VIII and should be considered if severe coagulopathy is present. It is given in a dose of 1 U/5 kg.
- Platelets should be given in a dose of 1 U/5 kg if the platelet count is less than $1,00,000/\mu L$. This will raise the platelet count by 50,000 µL. More liberal use is indicated in cyanotic patients because their platelets are usually dysfunctional.

Note: Platelet transfusions are not indicated in the patient who is not bleeding until the count falls below $30,000/\mu L$.

- Caution must be used when considering the transfusion of cryoprecipitate and platelets to patients with labile pulmonary hypertension. They can trigger an acute increase in pulmonary vascular resistance:
  - Add aprotienin—1.2 lakh kiu/m^2 over 1 hour, then 1.5 lakh kiu/m^2/h as infusion.

- Tranexamic acid—10 mg/kg over 1 hour, then 1 mg/kg/h as infusion.
- Fibrinogen (Elgen)—30 to 100 mg/kg qid, if fibrinogen levels are less than factor 7a—40 to 120 µg/kg.
- Desmopressin (DD AVP) 0.3 µg/kg IV in 50 mL normal saline over 20 minutes may be beneficial in cases of platelet dysfunction.
- Bleeding that continues despite normalization of coagulation studies often represents a mechanical source that warrants surgical exploration.

BLOOD PRODUCTS

Pump Blood

- It is the blood remaining in the cardiopulmonary bypass circuit on completion of bypass.
- It is a mixture of the patient's own blood, other fluids and any bank blood used to prime the bypass circuit.
- Pump blood has a low hematocrit and contains large amounts of heparin. The use of MUF (modified ultrafiltration) concentrates the pump blood to some extent and removes some heparin. If pump blood is used for volume expansion, additional heparin reversal will need to be given.
- It should not be used if excessive bleeding already exists or if the Hb is already inadequate.

Protamine Sulfate for Reversal of Heparin in Pump Blood

- Give 1 mg/25 mL of pump blood.
- Consider rechecking ACT after 10 mL/kg pump blood.

PACKED RED BLOOD CELLS (PRBC) (TABLE 7.1)

Uses

Used for treatment of anemia and the management of active bleeding.

TABLE 7.1: Content of a unit of PRBC.

Contents	
Unit	= 1 donation
Volume	280 ± 60 mL
Hematocrit	0.50–0.70
Sodium	20 mmol per unit (typically)
Potassium	0.5–5 mmol per unit (up to 15 mmol/L)

Warning: Neonates should be transfused with blood that is as fresh as possible, and sufficiently slowly to minimize any adverse effect from hyperkalemia and citrate toxicity (hypocalcemia).

Compatibility

Must be compatible with recipients ABO and Rh groups and clinically significant red cell antibodies.

Dose

- Transfusion of 4 mL/kg increases Hb by approximately 1 g/dL.
- In rapid transfusion situations, alternate red cell units with colloid solutions, e.g. FFP.

Notes

- Store only in a designated blood refrigerator (2–6°C).
- Use within 4 hours of removing from refrigerator.
- Always use a leukocyte filter.
- Request irradiated/products if suspicious of DiGeorge anomaly or previous intrauterine transfusion.
- Blood will uniquely expose the patient to transfusion-associated risks (infection, transfusion, reaction). Pump blood, however, is blood to which the patient has already been exposed.

PLATELETS

- Cardiopulmonary bypass frequently leads to both thrombocytopenia (dilutional) and more importantly platelet dysfunction (early onset).
- Platelet transfusion should be considered for excessive bleeding, irrespective of the absolute platelet count. (*see* below, for management of excessive bleeding).
- Platelet transfusion should not be used for "routine" volume expansion.
- *Dose:* 10 mL/kg—repeat platelet count.
- Should be ABO compatible to prevent hemolysis caused by donor anti-A and anti-B. Female infants and children (all females <45 years) should receive RhD negative platelets.
  Note: Transfused platelets also have a storage (function) defect lasting 2–4 hours.

FRESH FROZEN PLASMA

- Plasma separated from one donation of blood.
- Contains normal levels of stable clotting factors, albumin and immunoglobulin.
- Factor VIII levels are at least 70% normal.

Content

Slightly diluted plasma proteins including immunoglobulins and clotting factors.

Compatibility

It should be ABO compatible to prevent hemolysis caused by donor anti-A or anti-B.

Uses

- Treatment of microvascular bleeding following massive transfusion.
- Emergency reversal of coumarin anticoagulation. (give vitamin K also).
- Bleeding resulting from hepatic failure.
- Proven coagulopathy.

Dose

10–20 ml/kg IV.

Note

- Infection risk similar to other blood components.
- FFP transfusion should not be used for "routine" volume expansion.
- Loss of clotting factors may occur as a result of excessive loss of peritoneal, pleural fluid or ascites (via PD catheter). If replaced with NSA alone this may lead to a dilutional coagulopathy.

CRYOPRECIPITATE (CRYO)

Description

Cryoprecipitate is prepared from plasma and contains fibrinogen, von Willebrand factor, factor VIII, factor XIII and fibronectin.

Cryoprecipitate is available in pre-pooled concentrates of six units or singly. Each unit from a separate donor is suspended in 15 mL plasma prior to pooling. For use in small children, up to 4 single units can be ordered. Each unit provides about 350 mg of fibrinogen.

Indication

- Cryoprecipitate is indicated for bleeding or immediately prior to an invasive procedure in patients with significant hypofibrinogenemia (<100 mg/dL).
- Cryoprecipitate should not be used for patients with von Willebrand disease or Hemophilia A (factor VIII deficiency).
- It is not usually given for factor XIII deficiency, as there are virus-inactivated concentrates of this protein available.
- Cryoprecipitate is sometimes useful if platelet dysfunction associated with renal failure does not respond to dialysis.

▊HUMAN ALBUMIN SOLUTIONS

Supplied as 4% or 20% solutions (Table 7.2).

Composition

About 96% of the protein content of these solutions is albumin.

Note

- About 20% solution is hyperoncotic and in an ideal situation (i.e. normal capillary permeability) should expand circulating volume by a factor of 5. For every 10 mL infused, equivalent volume expansion occurs as would be seen with 50 mL iso-oncotic colloid (4% albumin).
- Hypotension has been reported in patients on ACE inhibitors who are given albumin.

Dosage

- Calculated on the basis that 1 unit/kg of factor VIII leads to a rise in plasma factor VIII of approximately 2%. Example: 50 units/kg will increase factor VIII level by ~ 100%.
- Doses are rounded up to the nearest vial size.
- The half life of factor VIII is 8–12 hours.

Administration

Factor VIII is generally administered as a slow bolus intravenous injection. Continuous infusion of factor VIII is indicated for patients requiring admission for severe bleeds or surgical procedures. Factor VIII replacement for such patients should be managed in consultation with the hemophilia unit or the hematologist on call. A continuous infusion of 3 units/kg/hour via syringe pump is commenced after a bolus loading dose.

Recombinant Factor VIII

- Genetically engineered factor VIII.
- The product of choice for the prevention and treatment of bleeding associated with hemophilia A (factor VIII deficiency).

TABLE 7.2: Human albumin.

4% Human albumin	20% Human albumin
Protein: 40 g/L	Protein: 200 g/L
Na: 140 mmol/L	Na: <140 mmol/L
Volume expansion	Hypoproteinemic edema
50 and 500 mL bottle	20 mL bottle
5–10 mL/kg aliquots	2–4 mL/kg aliquots

- It does not contain von Willebrand factor and is not indicated for the treatment of bleeding in von Willebrand's disease.

CARDIAC TAMPONADE

- Cardiac tamponade occurs when a collection of fluid (usually blood) around the heart, and usually within the pericardial space, compresses the heart chambers causing hemodynamic embarrassment.
- This is postoperative emergency and should be suspected when the following happen:
  - A fall in systemic blood pressure is accompanied by tachycardia and increased filling pressures.
  - Low cardiac output occurs in the presence of a tendency toward equalization of the left and right atrial pressures (even if these remain low).
  - Reduction or cessation of urine output occurs.
  - Decrease or cessation of chest drainage occurs, especially when this was previously large.
  - Widened mediastinal shadow on chest X-ray is observed.
  - Pulsus paradoxus (look at arterial waveform) (gentle pressure on chest may accentuate the paradox) is observed.
  - Echocardiographic evidence of pericardial collection is noted.
  - Dropping Hb despite packed cell volume (PCV) transfusion is observed.
  - Cardiac arrest occurs.
- A similar clinical syndrome can occur without a significant collection of mediastinal fluid (dry tamponade). This occurs due to the combined effect of mediastinal edema, intrathoracic pressure and a poorly functioning heart. An 'open chest' strategy may improve myocardial function until recovery occurs.

Note: Gauge piece packing may block tube and cause tamponade. Too much negative suction on drains gives a picture like tamponade.

Note: Absence of obvious collection on 2D echo or widened mediastinum on chest X-ray does not exclude cardiac tamponade.

Treatment: Arrange for immediate re-exploration of chest and inform the consultant intensivist and surgical team on call.

Chapter 8

Capillary Leak Syndrome

Prashant Shah

INTRODUCTION

Definition

Capillary leak syndrome typically develops in young patients who have undergone complex cardiac surgery, involving long periods of cardiopulmonary bypass or circulatory arrest, and who sustain periods of low cardiac output perioperatively. A similar clinical syndrome is seen in severe sepsis and other types of critical illness associated with systemic inflammatory responses.

The syndrome is thought to arise through the stimulation of inflammatory cascades, which results in damage to the capillary endothelium. "Leaky" capillaries disrupt the normal balance of oncotic and hydrostatic forces, as albumin and other large molecules are no longer reliably maintained within the capillary. Thus, proteins and fluids leak into the interstitium, further degrading the balance of forces across the capillary.

Features

- Unstable circulation with falling systemic pressure.
- Usually high inotrope requirement.
- Low filling pressures.
- Increased colloid requirement to keep filling pressures high.
- Absence of bleeding to explain the need for the colloid infusion.
- Increasing systemic edema, effusions, ascites, etc.
- Often low diastolic BP.

Who is at Risk?

- Neonates, infants after a prolong cardiopulmonary bypass, especially with circulatory arrest. Capillary leak is occasionally seen in very sick older patients.

When Does it Present?

It presents within 24 hours of cardiopulmonary bypass.

Management

There is no specific treatment for capillary leak. Management is aimed at supporting compromised systems:
- Keep the filling pressures as low as is compatible with good cardiac output.
- *Ventilation:* Pulmonary compliance deteriorates as interstitial edema and pleural effusions accumulate. Thus, higher ventilatory pressures are needed and increased levels of positive end-expiratory pressure (PEEP) may be needed to improve oxygenation.
- Optimize hemodynamics.
- There is some evidence that maintaining a high-normal hematocrit may help.
- Consider peritoneal drainage of ascitic fluid ± peritoneal dialysis if renal replacement therapy is indicated.
- Drainage pleural effusion may also be necessary/beneficial—improves lung mechanics, lowers right atrial pressure (RAP).
- Role of steroid is controversial but can be used in small dose.

Chapter 9

Cardiac Arrhythmias

Karthik Surya, Yogesh C Sathe

INTRODUCTION

Maintenance of normal sinus rhythm and atrioventricular synchrony is of paramount importance in every post-cardiac surgical patient. However, arrhythmias are a constant threat and need to be addressed with diligence, as proper identification is necessary for optimal management in these patients.

Postsurgical changes are one of the most important cause of arrhythmias secondary to resection or manipulation of ventricular or atrial tissues. Numerous nonsurgical causes are also seen and the total incidence of arrhythmias is 15 to 30% of all patients admitted in cardiac intensive care unit.

COMMON TYPES AND CAUSES OF ARRHYTHMIAS

Supraventricular arrhythmias:
- Junctional ectopic tachycardia [ToF repair, ventricular septal defect (VSD) surgical closure].
- Atrial tachycardia/atrioventricular nodal reentry tachycardia (balloon atrial septostomy, atrial cannulation, suture lines in atrium).
- Sinus bradycardia/low atrial rhythm (SA node injury, hypoxia, hypothermia).
- Sinus tachycardia (hyperthermia, excessive catecholamines).

Ventricular arrhythmia (myocardial ischemia or disease due to any cause):
- Isolated premature ventricular beats (PVC).
- Multifocal PVCs.
- Ventricular tachycardia.
- Ventricular fibrillation.

Second and third degree AV block (sutures in area of bundle of His, VSD closure, subaortic resection).

Right bundle branch block (RBBB) (after surgeries on the RV).

Left bundle branch block (LBBB) (After left ventricular outflow tract surgeries).

Normal ECG as shown in Figure 9.1.

GENERAL APPROACH TO ECG

- Locate the P wave:
  - Distinct wave, flutter, fibrillation, retrograde, absent.
  - P wave axis.
  - High right atrium.
  - High left atrium (situs inversus).
  - Low left atrium.
  - Low right atrium (coronary sinus).
- Determine relationship of P wave to the QRS complex.
- Assess the R–R interval:
  - Regular (vary by less than 0.08 s).
  - Irregular.
  - *Rate:* Normal, low, high.
- *Measure the QRS duration:* Normal or prolonged.

SINUS BRADYCARDIA

- P wave precedes each QRS complex.
- P wave axis is normal for age.
- Normal rates for age:

<3 years	70–180
3–5 years	60–150
5–9 years	60–130
9–12 years	50–100
12–16 years	50–100

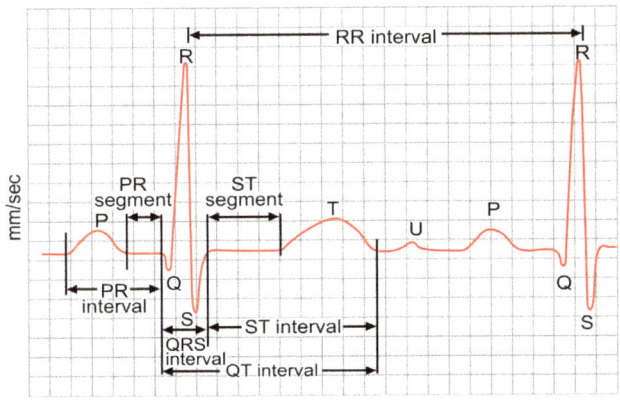

mm/mV 1 square = 0.04 sec/0.1 mV

Fig. 9.1: Normal ECG.

SINUS ARRHYTHMIA

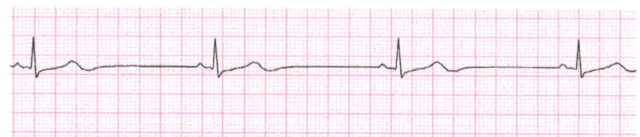

- Irregular discharge from sinus node—vagal influence.
- *Respiratory variation:* Decrease rate at end expiration.
- P wave precedes each QRS complex.
- Constant P wave axis.
- May have atrial premature beat (APB) or ventricular premature beat (VPB) in slow phase if intrinsic rate of subsidiary pacemaker exceeds slowest sinus rate.
- Normal in children and adolescents.

SUPRAVENTRICULAR TACHYCARDIA

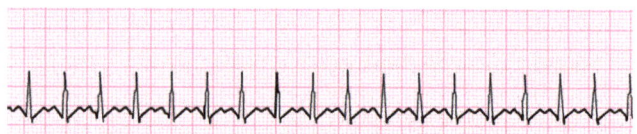

- Tachycardia resulting from abnormal mechanism arising proximal to the His bundles and which does not have morphology of atrial flutter.
- Most common symptomatic arrhythmia in children.
- *Ventricular rate*—mean 240:
  - *QRS complex narrow:* 92%.
  - *P wave detectable:* 56%.
  - *P wave axis:* Normal 15% (most common: 0-90°).
  - *WPW:* 22%.
- *Age of onset:*
  - 26% less than 1 month.
  - 34% less than 3 months.
  - 43% less than 1 year.
- *Less than 4 months:*
  - Increased incidence of congestive heart failure (CHF).
  - Decreased incidence of congenital heart defect.
  - Increased incidence of Walff-Parkinson-White (WPW).
  - Increased incidence of spontaneous remission.
- *Recurrence if untreated in infancy:* At least one more episode in 85%.
- *Congenital heart lesions:* Ebstein's malformation, L-TGA, postoperative—mustard, atrial septal defect (ASD) closure.
- Treatment:
  - *Acute:*

- If CHF:
  - Adenosine 0.05–0.25 mg/kg IV bolus.
  - *Rapidly metabolized:* Can repeat dose in 2–3 mintues.
  - *DC cardioversion:* 0.25–1.0 Ws/kg.
- *Vagal maneuvers:*
  - Ice bag to face, press on abdomen:
    - Valsalva maneuver, carotid sinus massage.
    - Successful in median age, 8.2 years.
  - Overdrive atrial pacing (intracardiac, transesophageal).
  - *Injection Amiodaron:* 5 mg/kg over 1 hour followed by 5 µg/kg/min and increased up to 25 µg/kg/min.
  - *Digoxin:* 20 mg/kg/IV; maximum 500 mg. Median time to cessation: 6 hours. Use with caution in WPW.
  - *Verapamil:* 0.1 mg/kg over 30–60s. Do not use in the presence of beta blocker, in patients less than 1 year of age, or for atrial fibrillation or atrial flutter associated with WPW as ventricular response rate may increase.
- *Chronic*—treat at least 1 year from last episode:
  - *Digoxin:* 10 mg/kg/day—suitable for infants.
  - Beta blocker:
    - *Inderal:* 1–7 mg/kg/day Q6-Q8.
    - *Atenolol:* 1–1.5 mg/kg/QD.
    - Type 1 or type 3 agents.
    - Radiofrequency ablation.

ATRIAL FLUTTER

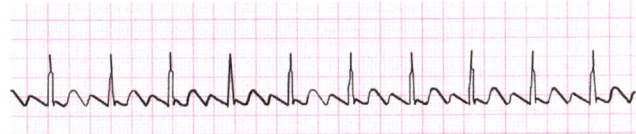

- Rapid atrial depolarizations, "sawtooth" 2,3, aVF.
  - *Atrial rate:* 280–450.
  - *Ventricular rate variable:* AV block 1:1 to 8:1, 2:1 common.
- High incidence of congestive heart failure.
- Treatment:
  - *Symptomatic:* Overdrive atrial pacing (intracardiac or TE).
  - *DC cardioversion:* 0.5–1.0 J/kg.
  - *Digoxin:* Increases AV block, slows ventricular response.
  - Digoxin followed by quinidine or other type 1 agents. Give digoxin first since quinidine facilitates AV

conduction; decrease maintenance digoxin dose by 50% if quinidine is used:
- Beta-blocker.
- Type 3 agents.
- Radiofrequency ablation.

ATRIAL FIBRILLATION

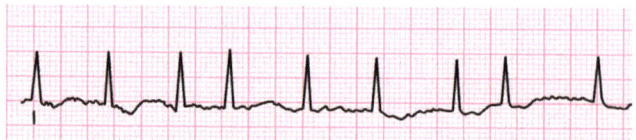

- Irregularly, irregular rhythm.
- *No definite P wave identifiable:* Wavering baseline.
- Older patients with severe rheumatic disease, Ebstein's anomaly, tricuspid atresia, ASD, cardiomyopathy, atrial tumor, Fontan procedure.
- Treatment if it causes hemodynamic changes significantly:
  - *Acute:* DC cardioversion:
    - Type 1 or type 3 agents combined with digoxin.
  - *Chronic:* Digoxin slows ventricular response.
  - Anticoagulate prior to cardioversion if concerned about the possibility of intracardiac clot. May need transesophageal echocardiogram.

JUNCTIONAL ECTOPIC TACHYCARDIA/HIS BUNDLE TACHYCARDIA

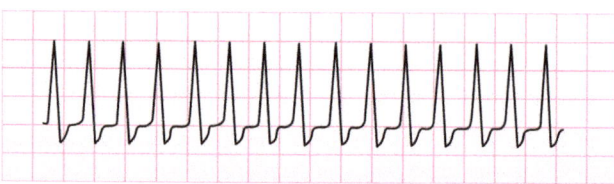

- Affects 2 to 5% of postsurgical patients.
- *Cause:* Surgical manipulation near AV node area, improper stretch or pull of tricuspid valve for retraction.
- At risk patients—post-tetralogy of Fallot correction; postsurgical VSD closure.

Characteristics

- Impulses arising at or near AV node.
- Discharge rate faster than atrial rate.
- Rates are usually accelerated above 180/min (140–220 bpm) with severe hemodynamic deterioration (hypotension and poor cardiac output).

- QRS complex identical to sinus rhythm, AV dissociation and occasional sinus capture beats.
- Will not respond to adenosine.

Treatment
- Early institution of cooling to 34°C centrally cornerstone of management.
- Amiodarone infusion—pretreatment with calcium chloride blunts the alpha blocking effects of amiodarone and prevents cardiovascular collapse from hypotension particularly in neonates and unstable patients.
- Pace atria to provide AV synchrony (overdrive pacing).
- Correct any electrolyte imbalance aggressively.
- Consider to reduce inotropes.
- Tab Ivabradine 0.1 mg/kg/day in 2 divided dose is firstline of managenet for JET.

WOLFF-PARKINSON-WHITE SYNDROME

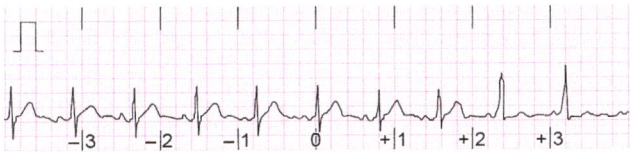

- *Short PR interval:*
  - ≤2 years   <0.08 s
  - 2–10 years   <0.10 s
  - >10 years   <0.12 s
- Delta wave caused by early activation of one ventricle (or part of one ventricle) by conduction down a bypass tract. QRS complex prolonged by as much as the PR interval is shortened. The QRS complex is a fusion between conduction via bypass tract and His bundles.
- *Congenital heart disease:* Ebstein's anomaly, L-TGA.
- *Treatment:* Only if SVT or atrial fibrillation occurs. Digoxin may decrease antegrade effective refractory period of accessory pathway. Beta-blockers are often effective. Radiofrequency ablation can provide permanent cure.

VENTRICULAR PREMATURE BEATS (VPB)

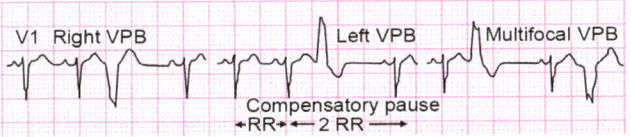

- QRS complex is premature, prolonged and of different morphology.

- *There are STT wave abnormalities:* T wave often opposite of normal.
- There is no preceding P wave.
- +Fusion beats.
- Usually full compensatory pause, but may interpolate.
- *Determine pattern:* Bigeminy, trigeminy, couples, uni- or multifocal.

VENTRICULAR TACHYCARDIA

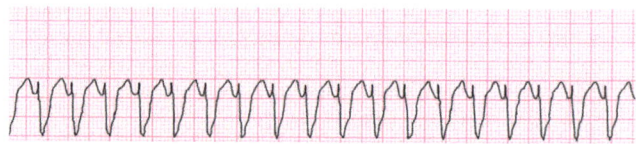

- Three or more consecutive VPBs.
- Wide QRS complex tachycardia:
  - *Differential diagnosis:* SVT with aberration (8% of SVT), atrial flutter with aberration.
- +AV dissociation can be detected.
- +Fusion beats.
- *Morphology often similar to single VPB:* Old ECG helpful.
- *Maximum rate:* 200–250 (rarely 270–300).
- Treatment:
  - Acute:
    - *Hypotension:* DC cardioversion—1.0–2.0 J/kg.
    - *Lidocaine:* 1 mg/kg IV bolus; 20–50 µg/kg/min infusion.
    - Overdrive ventricular pacing.
    - *Procainamide:* 5–10 mg/kg in 15–30 min—20–80 µg/kg/min infusion.
    - *Amiodaron:* 5 mg/kg IV bolus and 5–15 µg/kg/min infusion.
    - *Bretylium:* 5 mg/kg slowly over 15 min—20–50 µg/kg/min infusion.
    - *Dilantin:* 10 mg/kg over 30–60 min—5 mg/kg/day Q 12 hours.
  - *Chronic:* Beta-blocker, type 1 or type 3 agents, surgical or catheter ablation.

VENTRICULAR FIBRILLATION

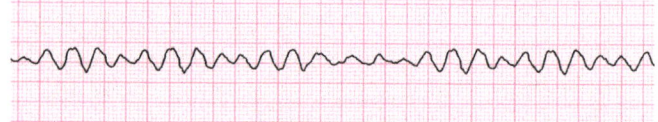

- Uncoordinated ventricular contraction without cardiac output.

- Low amplitude, rapid, irregular depolarizations without identifiable QRS complex.
- *Condition:* Prolonged QT syndrome, metabolic derangements, cardiomyopathy, WPW with short antegrade ERP of bypass tract.
- *Treatment:* DC cardioversion—1.0–2.0 J/kg.
- Management of hemodynamically significant arrhythmias has been described in Table 9.1.

FIRST-DEGREE HEART BLOCK (FIG. 9.2)

- *Prolonged PR interval:* Delay in AV node (common) or His-Purkinje.
- Each atrial impulse conducted to the ventricle.
- *Etiology:* Infection, congenital heart disease, medication (digoxin), hyperthyroidism, surgical trauma, high levels of vagal tone.
- *Treatment:* None needed.

SECOND-DEGREE HEART BLOCK (FIG. 9.2)

- Intermittent failure of conduction between atrium and ventricle.
- *Type 1 Wenckebach:*
  - Gradual lengthening of PR interval, gradual decrease of R-R interval, constant P-P interval.
  - *Treatment:* None needed unless medication related.
- *Type II:*
  - Constant PR, P-P intervals, nonconducted "conductable" P wave.

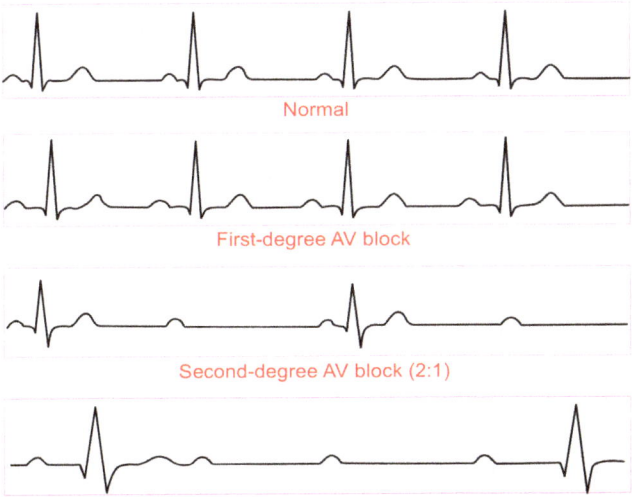

Fig. 9.2: ECG in conduction block.

TABLE 9.1: Drug therapy of acute hemodynamically significant arrhythmias in the cardiac intensive care unit (CICU).

Drug	Dose	Indications	Comments
Adenosine	100 µg/kg rapid bolus, double if ineffective, max 300 µg/kg	SVT	May cause sinus pauses bradycardia AV block
Amiodarone	Load 5 mg/kg over 30–60 min; may repeat × 2; infusion 15–20 mg/kg/24h	Atrial tachycardia, flutter, and fibrillation; JET; VT and VF	May cause sinus bradycardia; AV block, hypotension, drug interactions with procainamide and β-blocks
Atropine	10–20 µg/kg	Sinus bradycardia	
Epinephrine	1–5 µg/kg	Sinus bradycardia, AV block	
Esmolol	250–500 µg/kg load over 1–2 min 50–500 µg/kg/min infusion	Sinus tachycardia; atrial and ventricular tachyarrhythmias	May cause negative inotropy, bradycardia, sinus pauses AV block
Isoproterenol	0.01–0.03 µg/kg/min	Sinus bradycardia in denervated heart, complete AV block	effects may decrease diastolic BP
Lidocaine	1–2 mg/kg load over 1 min, may repeat, infusion 20–50 µg/kg/min	PVCs, VT, VF	Toxicity from hepatic/renal failure
Magnesium sulfate	25–50 mg/kg load over 30 min	VT (Torsade de pointes), prevention of JET	May cause muscle cramps
Procainamide	10–15 mg/kg load over 30–45 min; infusion 20–40 µg/kg/min	Atrial tachycardia, JET, VT	Monitor procainamide and N-acetylprocainamide levels may cause hypotension; synergistic adverse effects with amiodarone

(SVT: supraventricular tachycardia; AV: atrioventricular; JET: junctional ectopic tachycardia; VT: ventricular tachycardia; VF: ventricular fibrillation; PVC: premature ventricular contraction)

- *Block in His bundle:* 35%, below His bundle: 65%.
- *Treatment:* Acute with hypotension: isoprenalin, atropine; chronic: pacemaker.

THIRD-DEGREE HEART BLOCK (*SEE* FIG. 9.2)

- Atria and ventricles beat independently.
- Ventricular rate is usually slower than atrial rate.
- *Etiology:* L-TGA, maternal SLE, Lyme disease, surgical trauma.
- *Treatment:* Pacemaker if symptomatic (CHF, syncope, dizziness, exercise intolerance), ventricular rate <55 in infant, <40 in adult, >3 s pause in ventricular rate, block within or below. His bundle, greater than 2 weeks postoperatively.

Chapter 10

Care of the Patient with a Pacemaker

Yogesh C Sathe, Harun Ramasami

PACEMAKERS
- Provide repetitive electrical stimuli to the heart muscle in order to control the heart rate.
- Can be temporary or permanent.
- Consists of a pulse generator and electrodes (leads).

Temporary Pacemakers

Types
- Transcutaneous external pacemaker.
- Epicardial pacemaker.
- Transthoracic thoracic pacemaker.
- Transvenous endocardial pacemaker.

Indications
- Conduction disorders.
- Rate disorders.
- Prophylaxis.

Components
- Pulse generator (Fig. 10.1).
- Leads:
  - External.
  - Epicardial:
    - Transthoracic or transvenous.

Pacing Systems
- Unipolar.
- Bipolar:
  - Pacing cables.
- Black—negative, pacing terminal.
- Red—positive, ground terminal.

Insertion
- External—applied emergently at the bedside.
- Epicardial—leads are placed by the cardiac surgeon in the operating room.

Care of the Patient with a Pacemaker

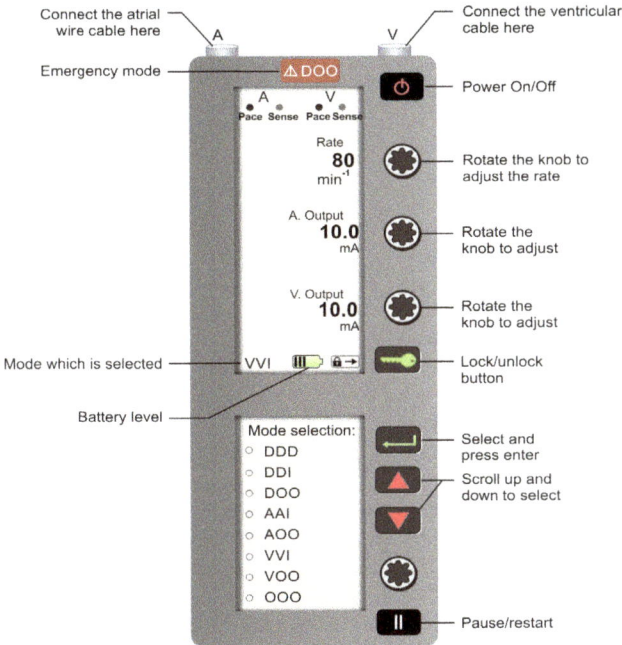

Fig. 10.1: Pacemaker display.

- Transthoracic—usually attempted emergently, as a last resort, after other temporary pacing methods have failed. A pericardial needle is inserted by the physician through the subxiphoid area of the thorax into the right ventricle and the lead wire is advanced through the needle to achieve contact with the endocardium.
- Transvenous—may be inserted at the bedside, preferably under fluoroscopy. Usually inserted into the subclavian or jugular vein, but can be inserted into the antecubital or femoral vein.

Settings

- *Rate:*
  - Fixed (asynchronous).
  - Stimulus is provided at a preset rate.
  - Rate is set greater than the patient's inherent rate to avoid competition.
  - Demand (synchronous).
  - Stimulus is provided when the patient's heart rate drops below at predetermined rate.
  - Must have adequate sensing.

- *Sensitivity threshold:*
  - Sensitivity.
  - Set in millivolts (mV).
  - Allows pacemaker to detect the patient's inherent R wave.
- *Sense indicator:*
  - Flashes when inherent R wave is detected.
  - Senses if pacing is in the demand mode.
- *Threshold:*
  - The minimum R wave amplitude needed to be detected by the pulse generator.
  - Once the sensitivity threshold is determined, the sensitivity is set 2–3 times lower.
- *Stimulation threshold:*
  - Output/mA:
    - Stimulus current is measured in milliamperes (mA).
    - Adjusted based on the amount of current needed to elicit myocardial depolarization and contraction. Variables—position of electrode; contact with viable myocardial tissue; level of energy delivered through wire; presence of hypoxia, acidosis or electrolyte imbalances and other medications being used.
  - Pace indicator:
    - Flashes each time a pacing stimulus is generated.
    - Does not necessarily indicate that a cardiac contraction occurred.
- *Pacing threshold:*
  - The minimum amount of mA's needed to achieve 100% capture.
  - The output is then doubled.

BASIC UNDERSTANDING OF DIFFERENT PACING MODES

By convention, pacing modes have four letters. But temporary pacemakers have only three:
- 1st letter stands for—chamber which is PACED (V: ventricle; A: atrium; D: dual).
- 2nd letter stands for—chamber which is sensed (V: ventricle; A: atrium; D: dual).
- 3rd letter stands for—mode of response (I: inhibit; T: trigger; D: dual response; O: no response).

For example:
- VVI (most commonly used):
  - 1st letter V indicates ventricular chamber is paced.
  - 2nd letter V indicates ventricular chamber is sensed.
  - 3rd letter I indicates inhibit response from the pulse generator. That means, if the patient's own beat

is generated, the pulse generator will not deliver impulse. It allows the native impulse of the heart to cause ventricular contraction.

Note: VVI mode is used if the pacing wire is kept on the ventricle.

- DDD:
  - 1st letter D indicates both chambers are paced.
  - 2nd letter D indicates both chambers are sensed.
  - 3rd letter D indicates dual response from the pulse generator. That means, the pulse generator either triggers an impulse or inhibits the impulse based on patient's own rhythm.

  Note: DDD is used when there are two pacing wires kept—one in atrium and another one in ventricle. This mode is closest to a physiological sinus impulse.

- VOO:
  - 1st letter V indicates ventricular chamber is paced.
  - 2nd letter O indicates no chamber is sensed.
  - 3rd letter O indicates no response from the pulse generator. That means, the pulse generator will not deliver any response. Here the ventricle will be paced continuously irrespective of patient's own rhythm.
  - As described above the various other methods (DDI, DOO, AAI, AOO and AOO) also represent the same.

Pacing Modes

- Atrial asynchronous pacing—atrial fixed pacing:
  - Impulse initiated via the atria.
  - Pathway similar to normal conduction.
  - Can be initiated via epicardial atrial leads.
  - Can result in competition.
  - Used for asystole or symptomatic sinus bradycardia.
  - Contraindicated for atrial fibrillation or flutter and for persons with conduction delays.
- Ventricular synchronous pacing—ventricular demand pacing:
  - Impulse sent to the ventricle when the patient's inherent rate drops below the preset rate on the pulse generator.
  - No harmony between the atria and the ventricle.
  - Used as a backup system for sinus bradycardia, heart blocks, atrial fibrillation/atrial flutter with SVR and junctional rhythm.
- AV sequential asynchronous pacing—dual chambered fixed rate pacing:
  - Impulses sent to atria and ventricle at a predetermined rate and at a predetermined AV interval regardless of patient's own rhythm.
  - Normal conduction through the heart.

- Used for asystole, symptomatic sinus bradycardia and for varying degrees of heart block to maintain AV conduction.
- AV sequential synchronous pacing—dual chambered demand pacing:
  - Impulses sent to atria and ventricles when the patient's rated drops below the preset rate on the pulse generator.
  - Normal conduction through the heart.
  - Used for asystole, symptom symptomatic sinus bradycardia and heart block.

Special Considerations

- Epicardial pacing:
  - Connect the negative pacing terminal to the epicardial lead electrode that is attached to the heart chamber to be paced.
  - Connect the positive ground terminal to another epicardial lead electrode, subcutaneous pacing wire, subcutaneous needle or skin patch electrode.
  - Determine sensitivity threshold and pacing threshold.
  - Set pacemaker settings.
  - Initiate pacing.
  - Be sure to follow hospital policy and protocol for initiating and adjusting pacemaker settings.

Troubleshooting

- Failure to fire—cannot see pacemaker spikes during periods of asystole or bradycardia:
  - Loose connections in the pacing system.
  - Failure of pacemaker battery or pulse generator.
  - Fracture of the pacing lead wire.
  - Lead wire dislodgement.
- Failure to capture—pacemaker spike is not followed by a P wave or QRS as appropriate:
  - Loose connections in the pacing system.
  - Increased pacing threshold.
  - Fracture of the pacing lead wire.
  - Lead wire dislodgement.
  - Failure of pacemaker battery or pulse gene.
- Undersensing—pacemaker fires with no regard to the patient's own rhythm. This is dangerous because it may lead to ventricular tachycardia and/or ventricular fibrillation:
  - Inadequate QRS signal.
  - Myocardial ischemia, fibrosis, electrolyte imbalances, bundle branch block, or a poorly positioned lead.

- Oversensing—pacemaker thinks it detects a QRS complex, inhibits itself and does not fire.
- Tall or peaked P waves or T waves.
- Myopotentials (electrical signals produced by skeletal muscle contraction as with shivering or seizures).

PATIENT MANAGEMENT

- ECG monitoring.
- Hemodynamic monitoring.
- Assessing pacemaker function.
- Electrical safety.
- Reassessing functioning after defibrillation.
- Pacing insertion site care.
- Assuring pacemaker controls are protected from accidental adjustment.
- Providing information regarding pacemaker therapy to the patient and family.

Chapter 11

Chest Drain: Care, Insertion and Removal

Amit Mishra

CHEST TUBES: CARE, INSERTION AND REMOVAL

Following cardiac surgery, drainage tubes are placed in the:
- Mediastinum.
- Pericardium.
- Pleural cavity.

All are drained into glass bottles with underwater seal. The underwater seal tube should not touch the bottom of the bottle.

Objectives: To drain blood, fluid and air.

MANAGEMENT OF TUBES

- Low-pressure suction to be applied to all tubes from low-pressure suction machine (10–20 cm H_2O) at the side port of the suction bottle.
- Tubes to be milked regularly if blood drainage is thick and associated with clots.
- Drainage to be measured and watched for any excess drainage of blood for proper management. Blood loss greater than 10 mL/kg/h suggests excess bleeding; surgeon to be informed (*see* Chapter 7).
- If tubes have to be clamped, clamps to be removed as quickly as possible.
- All tubes to be surrounded with sterile dressing to avoid infection.
- Chest X-ray to be obtained if drainage is excessive or suddenly stops.

REMOVAL OF TUBES

- Progressive fall in and cessation of drainage.
- Blocked tubes refractory to milking.
- Expansion of lung with stoppage of air bubble fluid from pleural space.
- During chest drain removal inform patient to take deep breath and hold it.

Chest Drain: Care, Insertion and Removal

- For small babies, tubes can be removed during inspiration.
- In this way, we should prevent AIR SUCK into chest cavity.
- Pain to be mitigated during removal with analgesic/sedative.
- Pericardial tube is removed first, followed by mediastinal tube.
- Sterile dressing of site to be done after removal of tube.
- Chest X-ray to be obtained after removal.

INSERTION OF INTERCOSTAL CATHETERS

Objectives

To decompress pleural space and relieve respiratory distress.

The tube site is fifth space in the mid axillary line, at the upper border of the lower rib, directed toward the suprasternal notch (Fig. 11.1).

Equipment

- As for needle aspiration plus, argyl/portex catheter.
- Scalpel blade, artery forcep, needle holder, tissue forcep.
- Suture material silk, sterile towel, glove.
- Tube connector and under water seal.
- Drainage bottle.
- Low suction apparatus.

Procedure

- Scrub well and put on sterile gloves.
- Prepare skin well with betadine over a wide region around the catheter site.
- Inject local anesthetic up to pleura (Fig. 11.2).
- Make skin incision at the identified catheter site of insertion.
- After making a track for the catheter through the skin incision, introduce the catheter held on to the

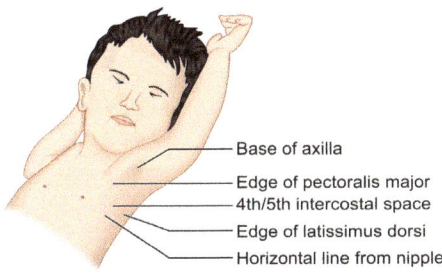

Fig. 11.1: Site of insertion.

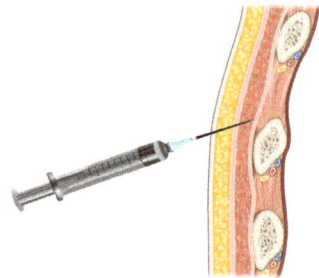

Fig. 11.2: Local anesthesia.

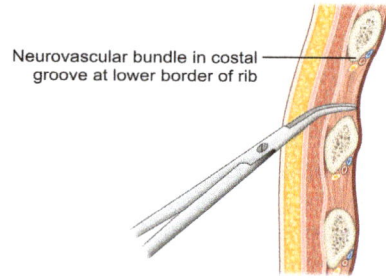

Neurovascular bundle in costal groove at lower border of rib

Fig. 11.3: Dissection with artery forceps.

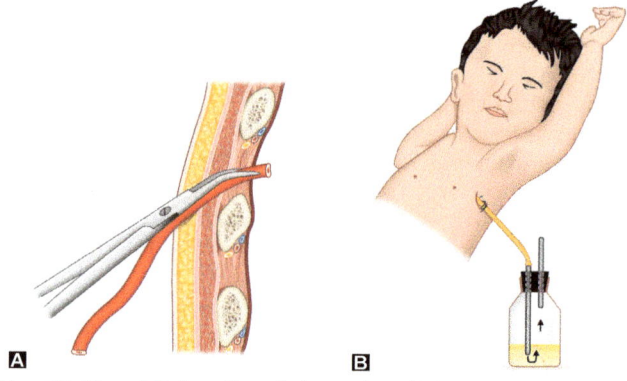

Figs. 11.4A and B: Insertion of chest tube with help of artery forceps.

tip of an artery forcep by firm but gentle rocking movements upward and medially into the pleural space (Figs. 11.3 and 11.4).
- Connect the catheter to the underwater seal bottle.
- Secure the catheter with suture to the skin.
- Place dressing surrounding the catheter.

Chest Drain: Care, Insertion and Removal

- Apply elastoplasts over the dressing to ensure an airtight seal and support the weight of the tubing. Avoid kinking of the tube.
- Check for drainage of air/fluid in underwater seal and swing with respiration.
- Connect low suction apparatus.
- Check whether connections are airtight and underwater seal tube does not touch the bottom of the bottle.
- Obtain chest X-ray to look for re-expansion of lung and position of the IC tube.

PLEURAL FLUID ASPIRATION

Objective

Removal of intrapleural collection of fluid if it is considered significant and impairs respiratory function, causing respiratory distress. Pleural fluid is suspected by physical signs over the chest and confirmed by X-ray.

Equipments

- Sterile tray containing aspiration set comprising stainless steel bowl.
- Artery clamps.
- Sterile gauze pieces.
- Sterile skin towels.
- Betadine for skin preparation.
- *Lignocaine:* 2% for local anesthesia.
- *Sterile disposable syringes:* 5 mL, 10 mL, 20 mL, 50 mL.
- Three-way stop cocks.
- 22G, 20G needles.
- Sterile bottle to collect aspirate and measure.
- Sterile vials for biochemistry and microbiology culture and antibiotic sensitivity.
- Sterile gloves.

Procedure

- Scrub well and wear gloves.
- Identify puncture site (7–9 space in midaxillary line) and prepare the regional skin with betadine.
- Inject lignocaine 1% at the puncture site superficial to pleura with 22G needle fitted to 5 mL syringe to induce local anesthesia. Insert 20G needle fitted to 20 mL/50 mL syringe through a three-way stopcock slowly at the upper edge of the rib using gentle suction with syringe until fluid is aspirated.
- Withdraw fluid until aspiration becomes difficult and little or no fluid is drawn.
- Collect fluid in the sterile bottle and measure.

- Send fluid specimen for biochemistry and culture and sensitivity, if exudates are suspected.
- Cover puncture site with sterile dressing.
- Obtain chest X-ray following aspiration.
- Monitor patient clinically and hemodynamically during the procedure.
- Ensure that no air is drawn into the pleural space during the procedure.

Chapter 12

Feeding and Nutrition

Shrishu Kamath, Lakshmi M

INTRODUCTION

Adequate nutrition is an important aspect in the management of a critically-ill child. Nutritional support is vital for minimizing the catabolic effects of stress of surgery and ensuring a positive nitrogen balance for tissue repair. The average caloric requirement in the postoperative period ranges from 120 to 150 kcal/kg.

Substrate mix
- Protein—20% of total calories.
- Carbohydrates—60–70%.
- Fats—20–30%.

Enteral Nutrition

Enteral feeding whenever feasible is the preferred route of administering nutritional support in a functioning gut. It corrects the pH of the gut, reduces bacterial overgrowth, preserves gut barrier function and minimizes the delay in gastric emptying.

The presence of bowel sounds and passage of flatus/stool are not prerequisites to initiate enteral feeds. In the absence of absolute contraindications, enteral feeds are initiated 2 hours after extubation. Care should be exercised in patients following repair of aortic coarctation in whom there may have been some degree of peroperative gut ischemia/reperfusion. Children with aortic coarctation are not normally fed by mouth until the day after surgery.

Nasogastric (NG) feeding is resorted to in ventilated patients. Feed are withheld 4 hours prior to a planned extubation.

Enteral feeds are initiated with an initial rate of 1 mL/kg per hour after documenting a baseline abdominal girth. Feeds are administered every 2 hours. We do not routinely aspirate gastric contents before each feed. It is done only if the abdominal girth increases by over 2 cm from the baseline. In such an instance, feeds are withheld if the pre-feed aspirate exceeds 50% of feed volume.

Steps of intragastric tube feeding:
- Before starting a feed, check the position of the tube.
- Remove the plunger of a sterile syringe and connect the barrel of the syringe to the end of the gastric tube.
- Pinch the tube and fill the barrel of the syringe with the required volume of feed.
- Elevate the syringe barrel and let the feed run through by gravity.
- Control the flow by altering the height of the syringe. Lowering the syringe slows the flow. Raising it hastens the flow.

Prokinetics with histamine-2-receptor antagonist (H2RA) or a proton pump inhibitor (PPI) are used in infants with gastroesophageal reflux.

Prokinetic agents
- Domperidone (0.1 mg/kg/dose TDS).
- Metoclopramide (0.1–0.3 mg/kg/dose TDS/QID).
- Cisapride (0.2 mg/kg/dose TDS/QID).
- *H2RA*—Ranitidine (8 mg/kg/day in 2 divided doses).
- *PPI*—Omeprazole (1 mg/kg/day in 2 divided doses).
- Lansoprazole (15 mg OD—less than 30 kg, 30 mg OD-more than 30 kg).

Parenteral Nutrition

If a patient is not receiving reasonable calories by the second postoperative day or the nutritional route in inaccessible for any reason, parenteral nutrition should be considered and the "Guidelines for the provision of total parenteral nutrition (TPN) to Cardiac Patients" consulted. The dietician should be involved in assessing nutritional intake:
- Consider TPN in postoperative ileus, gut ischemia and malabsorption.
- Use amino acids, glucose, trace elements, minerals vitamins and lipid emulsions.
- Nitrogen requirements are generally met by crystalline amino acid solutions.

Dosing guidelines
Aminoven—start with 1–1.5 g/kg/day. Increase by 1 g/kg/day to a maximum of 3.5 g/kg/day (Table 12.1).

TABLE 12.1: Age-related protein requirements.

Age	Protein (g/kg/day)
Term infant	2.0–2.5
Older infant	2.5–3.0
Older child	1.5–2.5

Intralipid—start with 0.5-1 g/kg/day. Increase by 0.5 g/kg/day to a maximum of 4 g/kg/day. Delivered separate from the infusate containing amino acids and glucose.

Carbohydrates—start with glucose infusion rates (GIR) of 4-6 mg/kg/min. Once the GIR supports acceptable serum glucose values, it is advanced gradually in a stepwise fashion (0.5-1 mg/kg/min) up to 8-10 mg/kg/min. A glucose concentration >12.5% must be delivered through a central vein:
- Vitamins—MVI 1.5 mL/kg.
- Trace elements—celcel.
- Intake of electrolytes and minerals has been described in Table 12.2.

Monitoring a patient on TPN
- Blood sugar-2-3 times a day while increasing GIR. Once a day when on a stable GIR.
- Serum albumin, Liver function tests, triglycerides, PCV, calcium, magnesium and phosphorus—once a week.

Prevention of infection
- Aseptic precautions during preparation of PN.
- Use of laminar flow.
- No compromise on disposables.
- No reuse of PN solutions.
- Use of bacterial filter in aminoven-dextrose line.

Complications of TPN
Hyperglycemia, hypoglycemia, electrolyte abnormalities, hypokalemia, hypophosphatemia, hypertriglyceridemia, cholestasis.

Minimal Enteral Nutrition

The practice of providing trophic feeds (small volume feeds with minimal calories) is considered a strategy to facilitate smooth transition from parenteral to enteral nutrition.

Recommended intake is 10-15 mL/kg/day, divided into equal aliquots and administered 3-6 hourly depending on tolerability.

TABLE 12.2: Recommended daily intake of electrolytes and minerals for TPN solutions.

Element	Requirement
Sodium	2-4 mEq/kg
Potassium	2-3 mEq/kg
Chloride	2-3 mEq/kg
Magnesium	0.25-0.5 mEq/kg
Calcium gluconate	100-150 mg/kg
Phosphorus	1-2 mmol/kg

SUGGESTED READING

1. Ford EG. Nutritional support of pediatric patients. Nutr Clin Prac. 1996;11:183-91.
2. Heyland DK. Nutritional support in the critically ill patient. Crit Care Clin. 1998;14:423-40.
3. Norris KKG, Steinhorn DM. Nutritional management during critical illness in infants and children. Crit Care Med. 1981;9:580-3.

Chapter 13

Postoperative Pulmonary Subsystem Issues and Management

Sachin S Patil, Ajith Sunny

POSTOPERATIVE PULMONARY SUBSYSTEM PROBLEMS: UPPER AIRWAYS OBSTRUCTIONS

Stridor—postextubation subglottic edema:
- Subglottic stenosis (congenital/acquired).
- *Vocal cord dysfunction:* Laryngo/tracheomalacia.
- *Endotracheal (ET) tube complications:* Incorrect size or inadequate analgesia/sedation during weaning with a struggling infant leading on to subglottic trauma followed by edema. Injury to recurrent laryngeal nerve during surgery (COA, PDA), causing a transient/permanent left vocal cord paralysis.

MANAGEMENT

- It is essentially prevention.
- Avoid oversized ET tubes.
- Do not allow child to struggle on ventilator, keep the child adequately sedated.
- Before extubation, check for air leak. If there is no air leak, start initial dose of IV dexamethasone 0.15 mg/kg, 12 hours followed by the second dose 6 hours before extubation.
- Noninvasive continuous positive airway pressure (CPAP) may be considered.
- Adrenaline nebulisation every 2–3 hourly.
- Consider reintubation in case of poor air-entry, desaturation and child looking exhausted in spite of above measures.

REINTUBATION

- Smaller ET tube preferred.
- Nasal route preferred.
- Light T tube.
- Heavy sedation or neuromuscular blockade when on mechanical ventilation. Dexamethasone 0.5 mg/kg for every 6 hours until 24 hours after extubation.

- Extubation failure.
- Bronchoscopic evaluation, if failed twice, tracheostomy, laser.

PHRENIC NERVE LESIONS

- Diaphragmatic paralysis/paresis—due to insults as nerve transaction, nerve stretch, electrocautery trauma or cold injury from topical cardiac hypothermia.
- *Incidence:* Up to 10% in infants <2 years.
- Common after Blalock-Taussig (BT) shunt, Glenn procedure, PDA ligation and COA repair.

Phrenic nerve lesion should be suspected, whenever there is unexplained persistent atelectasis, paradoxic movement of abdomen, inability to wean from ventilator in early postoperative period. Difficult to diagnose clinically (particularly on one side, infant) because of chest tubes and assisted ventilation.

Progressive elevation of a hemidiaphragm on serial chest X-rays confirmed by fluoroscope/ultrasound during spontaneous breathing in nonventilated patient.

Most spontaneously resolve controversy over plication of diaphragm to appropriate timings in infants and young children.

Plication decreases the number of days on mechanical ventilation with possible extubation within 2-6 days of plication. Hence, early plication is advocated. Nevertheless, as spontaneous recovery is possible within 2-3 weeks, plication is indicated only if there is difficulty in weaning from ventilation within 2-6 weeks.

Depending on circumstances of phrenic nerve trauma (known mechanical trauma during cardiac surgery like Glenn) and failure to extubate on two occasions—plication should be considered early (postoperatively—1 week).

PNEUMOTHORAX

- Alveolar rupture (CP resuscitation, mechanical ventilation).
- Air can escape into perivascular space, travel along perivascular sheath, rupture into mediastinum and later into pleural space.
- Massive or continuous air leak can cause tension pneumothorax.
- Cardiorespiratory compromise with hypoxemia, hypercarbia, tachycardia, hypotension warrants swift decompression by insertion of chest tube in pleural space.
- Tube left in place for 2-3 days.

- Bronchopleural fistula (2–3 weeks).
- Pleurodesis or pleurectomy.

HYPOXIA AND ITS MANAGEMENT (TABLE 13.1)

TABLE 13.1: Hypoxemia and its management.

Causes	
Ventilation related	Interventional procedure and drug therapy
ET tube obstruction/malposition	Gentle suction/change position/reintubates if need be
Improper ventilator settings	Correct settings guided by ABG
Underlying disease problems	
Pneumothorax	Decompression by tube insertion
Atelectasis	Gentle suction, chest physiotherapy
Secretions, aspiration	Mucolytic, nebulization
Bronchospasm	Salbutamol/Ipravent nebulization
Pulmonary edema	Morphine, diuretic, per dialysis
Decreased cardiac output	Volume expansion, inotropes, vasodilators, and base corrections

PLEURAL EFFUSION

Transudate

- Increase in capillary hydrostatic pressure—CCF.
- Increase in right-sided cardiac pressure—venous hypertension.
- SVC obstruction and overhydration can result in transudate in pleural space.

Exudates

- Commonly due to increased capillary permeability from nonspecific inflammation acute respiratory distress syndrome (ARDS), or reperfusion injury, infection and pulmonary infarction.
- Progressive slow collection can be asymptomatic. Cardiorespiratory compromise warrants chest tube drainage.

CHYLOTHORAX

Definition

- It refers to the presence of lymphatic fluid in pleural space secondary to leakage from thoracic duct/tributaries.

Prevalence
- *After various cardiothoracic surgeries: 0.2–1%.*

Investigation
- Serum electrolytes, serum albumin level, complete blood counts to look for lymphocyte depletion need to be done specifically.
- Lymphangiography is useful when the anatomy of the thoracic duct needs to be defined preoperatively or when the site of leak is not clinically obvious.
- Pleural fluid analysis for triglyceride content helps to confirm diagnosis of chylothorax.
- At levels greater than 110 mg/dL, there is maximum likelihood that the fluid is chyle.
- A ratio of pleural fluid cholesterol to triglyceride of less than 1 is also diagnostic.
- Chylomicrons seen under microscopy is a confirmatory test.

Management
- Patient can be treated by conservative management or by surgery in resistant, prolonged cases.

Medical Management of Chylothorax
- Conservative management helps as thoracic duct closes spontaneously in nearly 50% of cases. Inter coastal tube drainage of chylothorax needs to be done.
- New chyle production is reduced by total parenteral nutrition (nil per orally for 48–72 hours) or a fat-restricted oral diet supplemented with medium-chain triglyceride.
- Somatostatin, or its analogue octreotide, has been reported successful in a number of cases of chylothorax at doses ranging from 3 to 10 µg/kg/h over 48–72 hours with nil per oral regimen.
- Diarrhea, hypoglycemia and hypotension are side effects of somatostatin therapy.

Surgical Management of Chylothorax
- Its timing is controversial and needs to be individualized as per etiology and patient condition.
- Indications for surgery:
  - Leak >1 L/day for 5 days or a persistent leak for >2 weeks despite conservative management.
  - Nutritional/metabolic complications.
  - Loculated chylothorax/fibrin clots/trapped lung.
- Available surgical options are as follows:
  - Thoracic duct ligation.
  - Pleuroperitoneal shunt.

- Pleurodesis.
- Surgical pleurectomy.
  Kindly refer Appendix A2.6 (chylothorax algorithm).

BRONCHOSPASM (WHEEZE)

Salbutamol
- *Nebulization mild:* Respiratory solution (5 mg/mL, 0.5%) 0.5 mL/dose diluted to 4 mL, every 3–6 hours; moderate: 0.5%, severe (in ICU) 1 mL/dose diluted to 4 mL, every 1–2 hours; 0.5% solution undiluted continuously.
- Budecort nebulizer—0.5 mL dil with saline q8–12 hours or Aminophylline infusion—0.5–1 mg/kg/h.

Ipratropium
- Respiratory solution (250 µg/mL) 1 mL diluted to 4 mL, every 4–6 hours (25 µg/kg).

Terbutaline
- *Terbutaline (severe refractory):* IV 5 µg/kg stat. over 10 minutes, then 1–10 µg/kg/h.
- *Terbutaline nebulizer:* 0.5 mL q4–6 hours.
- *Systemic steroid therapy:* Decadron 24 hours before extubation; continue × 6 hours.
- *Chest physiotherapy:* If secretions in airways.

Chapter 14

Postoperative Gastrointestinal Issues

Prashant Shah

PARALYTIC ILEUS

- Suspected when feeds are not tolerated.
- *Symptoms:* No stools/flatus/bowel sounds.
- Increasing abdominal distenstion.
- Management:
  - Abdominal X-ray to exclude any organic cause.
  - Glycerine suppository.
  - Correction of potassium if there is hypokalemia.
  - Feeds discontinued until bowel sounds return to normal and abdominal distension regresses.

STRESS ULCERS

- All patients have a nasogastric (NG) tube placed routinely prior to surgery.
- The NG tube is kept open to drain initially.
- Observe and document any upper gastrointestinal (GI) bleed:
  - Sucralfate is prophylactically administered to all patients postoperatively until feeds are commenced.
  - *Dose:* 0–2 years—250 mg; 3–12 years—500 mg; 12 years—1 g; for every 6–8 hours.
  - *Ranitidine*—1 mg/kg/dose every 6–8 hours IV:
    - Administered in cases of documented GI bleed and if child is on aspirin.
    - Frequency of drug is adjusted in presence of renal failure.
  - *Pantoprazole:* 1 mg/kg/day.
  - Oral antacids also used (especially if the patient is on aspirin or ibuprofen).

ICTERUS

- Jaundice is seen in 2–9% of patients in the early postoperative period with increased serum bilirubin, normal or increased serum enzyme levels.

- Initiate therapy in preterms with serum bilirubin, 8–10 mg, and term babies, above 10–12 mg.
- Avoid hepatotoxic drugs.
- Rule out cardiac problems, hemolysis, infection and act accordingly.

NECROTIZING ENTEROCOLITIS (NEC)

- *Owing to local ischemia:* Reported in patients under 1 year of age operated under deep hypothermic circulatory arrest (DHCA). Beware in all patients (preoperative and postoperative) who are premature or have diminished systemic perfusion/increased pulmonary perfusion.
- *Clinical signs:* Tender distended abdomen, hypoactive bowel sounds, black stools, sepsis.
- *Radiology:* Pneumatosis intestinalis, distended bowel loops, free air in portal vein, fluid levels in bowel loops.
- *Management*—nil per oral, NG drainage:
  - Large-volume infusions.
  - *Systemic antibiotics:* Aggressive therapy, against aerobic, anerobic and fungal organisms with microbiologic cultures.
  - Close monitoring for infarction/perforation, which may warrant surgery.
  - Prognosis is poor.

GASTROINTESTINAL BLEEDING

- *Stress ulcers:* Risk factors are cardiogenic shock, prolonged surgery and trauma.
- Relatively uncommon.
- Multiorgan failure, sepsis, congestive cardiac failure (CCF) and steroids increase risk.

Medical Therapy

- Antacids.
- H_2 *antagonists:* Ranitidine IV 1 mg/kg/dose slowly for every 6–8 hours or 2 µg/kg/min infusion.
- *Oral:* 2–4 mg/kg/min.
- *Oral:* 2–4 mg/kg/dose (maximum 300 mg) for every 12 hours.
- Cold saline wash through ryles tube.

Sucralfate

- Both as therapy and prophylaxis, drug of choice.
- Enteral feeds are protective.
- Endoscopy in refractory medical therapy.
- In multiorgan failure, prognosis worse.

Chapter 15

Postoperative Central Nervous System Issues

Shrishu Kamath, Lakshmi M

PROTOCOL FOR SEIZURES IN INFANTS AND CHILDREN

General Comments

- Neuroprotective physical interventions in cardiac surgery include:
  - Maintaining cerebral perfusion.
  - Reducing cerebral embolization.
  - Temperature management.
  - Acid-base management.
- A potentially significant yet rare complication of cardiopulmonary bypass is neurologic injury resulting in stroke or seizures.
- *Seizure etiologies include:* Metabolic; infectious; cerebral edema, embolism or hemorrhage; systemic/cerebral hypoperfusion.
- The initial evaluation is to identify possible correctable causes and describe an emergent treatment regimen.
- Respiratory arrest, discoordinate respiratory activity or sudden inability to adequately mechanically ventilate can be an indication of seizural activity in infants.
- After initial control of seizures, anticonvulsant therapy should be continued through the recovery period. Decisions regarding long-term therapy are made by the neurologist or pediatric cardiologist before hospital discharge.
- Most children having a seizure in the early postoperative period will not have a chronic seizure disorder.
- Choreiform movements are more serious symptoms than seizures and are more apt to persist.
- Because of its potential to cause cardiorespiratory depression and its short duration of action, diazepam (Valium) is best avoided as an anticonvulsant unless the patient is being artificially ventilated.

Initial Evaluation and Treatment

At the onset of a seizure, arterial blood gases and pH; serum glucose, serum electrolytes (Na, K, Ca, Mg); cardiac index; and body temperature are determined.

The following derangements are considered contributory to seizure activity and are promptly corrected as per standard guidelines:
- pH <7.25 or >7.50; $PaCO_2$ <25 mm Hg; PaO_2 <80 mm Hg; and base deficit >10–15 mEq/L.
- Serum glucose level <40 mg/dL in infants and <60 mg/dL in older children.
- Serum calcium level <7 mg/dL in infants and <8 mg/dL in older children.
- Serum sodium level <125 mEq/L.
- Cardiac index less than 2 L/min/meter sqare.
- Body temperature >38.6°C (>101.5°F).

Anticonvulsant Therapy

When seizures are first noted, steps are taken to terminate them or, if they are no longer present, to prevent their recurrence while the biochemical parameters are being determined. Secure airway. Optimize breathing, circulation and temperature:
- Give:
  - 0.1 mg/kg of IV lorazepam (or) 0.1–0.2 mg/kg of IV diazepam (or) PR diazepam 0.5 mg/kg or buccal/nasal/IM midazolam 0.2 mg/kg.
  - 20 mg/kg of phenobarbitone IV over 20 minutes as a loading dose. If seizures continue, repeat phenobarbitone in 10 mg/kg/dose aliquots till 40 mg/kg is reached.
  - If seizures are not controlled by these measures, administer phenytoin 20 mg/kg over 30 minutes. Repeat a dose of 10 mg/kg if seizure persists.
- If there has been spontaneous termination of seizure activity and prevention of recurrence is desired, omit step 1a and proceed to step 1b/1c.
- In case of refractory seizures, consider alternate drugs including IV valproate, levetiracetam, midazolam infusion, propofol/pentothal.
- Maintenance anticonvulsant therapy is instituted 12–24 hours after the loading dose depending on the choice of the drug used to abort the seizure.

SUGGESTED READING

1. Arrowsmith JE, Grocott HP, Reves JG, et al. Central nervous system complications of cardiac surgery. Br J Anaesth. 2000;84(3):378-93.

Chapter 16

Postoperative Renal Issues and Peritoneal Dialysis

Prashant Shah

RENAL SYSTEM AND PERITONEAL DIALYSIS

- Minimal expected urinary output is 0.5 mL/kg/h in a child and 1 mL/kg/h in infants and neonates.
- Check that the urinary catheter is not blocked or incorrectly positioned.
- Palpate for bladder, if bladder is full then flush catheter with 10 mL injection water.

The most frequent cause of postoperative renal failure is low cardiac output, which may be potentiated intraoperatively by hypoxia, acidosis, hypoglycemia, volume overload, hypothermia, arrhythmias and the administration of alpha-adrenergic agonists or high dose of dopamine. It is more frequent in newborns and infants, in cyanotic patients and after long bypass times.

Indices in renal failure

	Urine osmolarity (mosm)	Urinary sodium	FE_{Na}
Prerenal	>500	<20 mmol/L	<1
Intrinsic	<350	>20 mmol/L	>1

$$FE_{Na} = 100 \times \frac{Sodium_{uninary} \times Creatinine_{plasma}}{Sodium_{plasma} \times Creatinine_{uninary}}$$

Check urinary creatinine.

Management

- Optimize cardiac output.
- Fluid challenge test (forced alkaline diuresis):
  - *Fluid (NS):* 10 mL/kg.
  - *Injection sodabicarb:* 1 mEq/kg state.
  - *Frusemide:* 1 mg/kg IV stat.
- This dose may be repeated up to 5 mg/kg.
- Avoid nephrotoxic drugs and give antibiotics according to renal clearance.

PERITONEAL DIALYSIS

- The surface area of the peritoneum is proportionally greater relative to total body mass in children compared with adults. Therefore, peritoneal dialysis is usually more efficient in neonates and infants than in larger children and adults.
- Advantages of peritoneal dialysis compared with other forms of dialysis include the following:
  - Usually better tolerated hemodynamically.
  - Easier to initiate.
  - Does not require arterial or venous access.
  - Is more likely to be effective independent of the hemodynamic state.
- Disadvantages are related to septic and mechanical complications of the peritoneal dialysis catheter and that it may occasionally cause respiratory compromise.
- Relative contraindications to peritoneal dialysis include recent abdominal surgery (< 1 week); peritonitis from any cause, particularly necrotizing enterocolitis; uncorrected gastroschisis, omphalocele or diaphragmatic hernia; or the presence of a ventriculoperitoneal shunt.
- Preparations of dialysate are usually used (Baxter Healthcare corp, Deerfield, IL). Three concentrations of dextrose are available: 1.5, 2.5 and 4.25 g/dL. Dextrose solution concentration with each dialysis cycle.
- Initiated with 1.5 g/dL solution and later changed if needed.
- Warmed prior to administration, and heparin (200 U/L) is usually added to the peritoneal dialysate.
- Primary variables that can be adjusted are the volume of dialysate used per cycle (20–40 mL/kg) and the dwell time (length of time in each cycle the fluid is allowed to remain in the peritoneal cavity).
- A typical starting regimen would be 20 mL/kg/cycle. Each cycle would last 1 hour, with 15 minutes for drainage.
- These variables are adjusted if needed. If more rapid fluid removal is needed, then a more concentrated solution or more rapid cycles may be needed.
- Another regimen that is gaining favor for neonates is the "rule of ten": 10 mL/kg/cycle, 10 minutes infusion, 10 minutes dwell and 10 minutes drain.
- Patients with severe metabolic acidosis may require bicarbonate to be added to the dialysate.
- The development of hypokalemia is common, in which case potassium can be added to the dialysate.
- Hyperglycemia can be addressed by adding insulin to the dialysate. Frequent monitoring of fluid status and electrolytes is needed.

- *Peritoneal dialysis (PD) cycles:* 1 hour cycle; 2 or 4 hours cycle. For 1 hour cycle—10 minutes running in; 30-40 minutes dwell time; 10-20 minutes running out.
- The efficacy of the peritoneal dialysis system can be judged by observing the ease with which the dialysis fluid is both run in and run out. There should be a net increase in the fluid run out as opposed to that run in.
- *Fluid balance:* The PD negative balance replaces urine flow if the child is anuric.
- Overall output = [(PD output − PD input) + urine output + insensible losses].
- It is vital that the rate of fluid removal is adjusted to maintain adequate cardiac filling pressures to preserve cardiac output.
- If serum Na^+ becomes elevated, a "low sodium" dialysis fluid is available (Dialaflex 63) (sodium content = 130 mmol/L).

During peritoneal dialysis, it is essential that the following steps are taken care of:
- Accurate input/output records are maintained, and it is usually desirable to record dialysis input and output separately from other fluid charts.
- Patients on dialysis can usually continue with oral or NG feeding, but if this is not tolerated, total parenteral nutrition (TPN) should be employed.
- If possible, patient should be weighed on a daily basis while on dialysis.
- Abdominal girth at umbilical level should be measured on an hourly basis.

Hemofiltration: Hemofiltration is available on the unit, and decisions on which form of dialysis should be used is taken in consultation with the nephrology team and the consultant intensivist. At present, peritoneal dialysis is the first choice for most operative cardiac patients.

Chapter 17

Pain Management (Sedation and Analgesia)

Sapna Varma, M Gokulakrishnan

INTRODUCTION

Adequate sedation and management of postoperative pain is very important for the successful outcome following congenital cardiac surgery. Newer sedatives and analgesics have helped in fast tracking and shortening stay in the ICU.

PROPERTIES OF AN IDEAL SEDATIVE

An ideal sedative agent would:
- Have a rapid onset of action, be easy to administer.
- Be effective at providing adequate sedation in order to alleviate noxious stimuli, stress and anxiety, while minimizing the risk of adverse events.
- Achieve effective analgesia, anxiolysis.
- Allow rapid recovery after discontinuation.
- Lack drug accumulation with be no symptoms of dependence, tolerance or rebound.
- Have few adverse effects especially cardio-respiratoy and reduced risk of delirium and agitation.
- Interact minimally with other drugs.
- And last but not the least be inexpensive.

INDICATIONS

- To counter stress responses associated with pain following cardiac surgery and cardiopulmonary bypass.
- To facilitate mechanical ventilation.
- To prevent excessive movement which may cause the invasive lines or chest drains to be pulled out.
- To prevent any surges in pulmonary vascular resistance (PVR) in patients with labile pulmonary hypertension.
- Higher doses may be required when there is a delayed sternal closure.
- To prevent fatal tachycardia which can increase myocardial ischemia and cause low cardiac output state.
- To aid in procedures like placement of invasive lines, chest drains, pericardiocentesis, cardioversion, bronchoscopy, transesophageal echocardiography.

SEDATIVES

Benzodiazepines
- Have anxiolytic, anticonvulsant, hypnotic and amnestic properties.
- Appropriate doses provide excellent conscious sedation.
- Causes myocardial depression.
- Hence, to be used with caution in low cardiac output patients.

Diazepam
- Long-acting and half-life of 24 hours, so mainly used for premedication.
- Oral/rectal/IV (causes significant pain).
- Cautious use in liver dysfunction and hypotension.

Midazolam
- Short-acting.
- IV, IM, oral, rectal.
- Useful as continuous infusion.
- Useful for procedures in pediatric intensive care unit (PICU).
- Poor bioavailability from high first-pass metabolism in liver. Hence, high doses required.
- Withdrawal symptoms on prolonged administration.

Lorazepam
- *Long duration of action:* 4–8 hours.
- Elimination half-life is approximately 18 hours.
- Oral, IM, IV useful for term sedation.

DEXMEDETOMIDINE: NEWER SEDATIVE
- Potent and highly selective α-2 adrenoceptor agonist with sympatholytic, sedative, amnestic and analgesic properties.
- Quick onset and a relatively short duration of action, easily titrated.
- Unique "conscious sedation" (patients appear to be asleep, but are readily roused).
- Bolus doses to be avoided as it causes bradycardia and hypotension.
- Has cardioprotective, neuroprotective, renoprotective properties.
- Does not cause respiratory depression and hence can be safely infused through tracheal extubation and later noninvasive ventilation.
- Decreases duration of mechanical ventilation and hence used for fast tracking and early extubation.

- Safe in neonates and preterm babies with a wide safety margin.
- May help in treating tachyarrhythmias especially after tetralogy repair.
- Can be safely used in patients with high PVR.

ANALGESICS

Opioid

- Mainstay, also provide sedation during mechanical ventilation:
  - Useful for Tetspells.
- Cautious administration in neonates and infants, <3 months, because of increased risk of respiratory depression:
  - *Commonly used:* Morphine, fentanyl.
  - *Tolerance development:* Time and dose related.
  - Withdrawal symptoms avoided by tapering dosage after prolonged administration.

Morphine

- Gold standard against which other opioids are compared.
- Better sedative than synthetic fentanyl.
- IV by continuous infusion for constant analgesic level.
- Can cause hypotension in presence of limited hemodynamic reserve.
- Also causes histamine release, which can potentially increase PVR and pulmonary arterial hypertension (PAH) and decrease the rate occurrence of SVR.

Fentanyl

- Shorter duration of action than morphine.
- Generates less histamine release, hence less vasodilation and hypotension.
- Approximately 100 times more potent than morphine. Rapid penetration of blood brain barrier due to high lipid solubility.
- *Rapid onset of action:* Effects last 30–45 minutes.
- Blocks stress response in a dose-related fashion while maintaining both systemic and pulmonary hemodynamic stability.
- *Caution:* Patients with high circulating catecholamine levels (CCF, critical aortic stenosis) can become hypotensive after a bolus induction dose.
- Beneficial in patients with risk of PAH due to lack of histamine release.
- Idiosyncrasy and dose-related side effects on rapid bolus administration are glottic and chest wall rigidity.
- Management—naloxone/paralysis.
- Potent analgesic with limited sedative effects.

Ketamine

- Phenyl cyclidine derivative.
- Rapid onset and short duration of action, 10–15 minutes, with elimination half-life of 2–3 hours.
- Administered IV/IM/IV infusion; useful for most PICU procedures.
- Produces a type of catalepsy, often with open eyes with nystagmus and intact corneal reflexes.
- Avoided in intracranial hypertension as it dilates cerebral blood vessels.
- Relatively contraindicated in patients with seizure disorders.
- Tachycardia, with increased cardiac output and increased BP due to sympathomimetic action from central stimulation.
- Minimal effects on PVR; hence safe in PAH.
- Bronchodilator and hence useful in reactive airways.
- *Side effects:* Delirium, hallucinations and night mares; controlled with benzodiazepines; benzodiazepines simultaneously administered with ketamine in older children in homes in whom frequency of nightmares is higher.

MUSCLE RELAXANTS

- Commonly used:
  - To facilitate intubation.
  - For controlled mechanical ventilation.
  - In limited cardiorespiratory reserve to decrease myocardial work and O_2 demand.
- Drawbacks of prolonged paralysis:
  - Risk of prolonged ventilator support.
  - Delay of enteral nutrition.
  - Tolerance and prolonged muscle weakness.
  - Prolonged hospital stay and cost.

NONDEPOLARIZING MUSCLE RELAXANTS

- These are competitive antagonists, competing with acetyl choline for binding to receptors at motor endplate.
- Agents are classified according to duration of action.
- For most patients, long-acting is not required if adequate sedation and analgesia is ensured.
- Duration of action is increased by acidosis, hypercapnia, hypothermia, administration of aminoglycosides, furosemide and antiarrhythmics.
- Action can be antagonized by antiacetylcholine esterase drugs such as neostigmine, edrophonium and pyridostigmine.

Vecuronium

- *Action:* 30 minutes; safe in limited hemodynamic reserve.
- Suitable as continuous infusion.
- When combined with fentanyl, a significant bradycardia necessitating atropine.

Pancuronium

- *Onset of action:* 2-3 minutes; duration approximately 1 hour.
- Safe with limited hemodynamic reserve, though it causes a mild tachycardia, increase in BP and cardiac output secondary to its vagolytic effect.
- Does not release histamine.
- Continuous infusion not advised.

ROCURONIUM

- Rapid onset (60-90 sec), with intermediate duration of action (20-40 min).
- Hence, can be used for rapid sequence intubation.
- Causes tachycardia, can be safely used with fentanyl.
- Can be used as continuous infusion.
- Can be easily reversed with no residual muscular weakness leading to rapid recovery.

ATRACURIUM

- Intermediate onset (2-3 min) with short duration (15-20 min).
- Metabolized by Haffmans elimination, hence not dependent on liver and kidney for metabolism and excretion.
- Can be safely used in hepatic and renal dysfunction, no prolongation of effects seen.
- May cause tachycardia and hypertension due to histamine release when given as a bolus, safe as a continuous infusion.

CONCLUSION

As no ideal sedative has been found a combination of sedative and analgesic agents are used to maximize efficacy and also to reduce doses and hence side effects. Newer sedatives have helped in fast tracking patients and reducing patients stay in the ICU. Right drugs in the right dose in the right hands at the right time is the key for successful outcomes.

Chapter 18

Inotropes

Prabhu Mayesesavan, Prashant Prasanna Bhaskar

DOPAMINE

- Dose-dependent effects on adrenergic receptors:
  - *0.5–2 μg/kg/min:* DA 1 splanchnic and renal vasodilation.
  - *2–6 μg/kg/min:* DA 1, β1 inotropic.
  - *6–15 μg/kg/min:* β > α1 inotropic > vasopressor.
  - *15–25 μg/kg/min:* α1 > β1 vasopressor.

Indications

- Decreased cardiac output due to poor contractility.
- Decreased renal perfusion.
- Poor peripheral perfusion without significant hypotension after volume resuscitation.
- *Administration:* Rapidly metabolized; hence continuous infusion through central vein.
- *Adverse effects at high doses:* Tachycardia, arrhythmias, peripheral gangrene due to increased vasoconstriction, local infiltration and tissue necrosis.

EPINEPHRINE

- Dose-dependent agonist effects on β1, β2 and α1 receptors:
  - *0.05–0.3 μg/kg/min:* β1 β2 > α1 inotrope, mild vasodilator.
  - *0.3–2 μg/kg/min:* β1 = α1 inotrope and vasopressor.
  - *1 μg/kg/min and higher:* β1 = α1 before finally α1 dominates over β1.

Indications

- Cardiogenic shock with collapse and myocardial dysfunction.
- Mandatory following CP resuscitation from cardiac arrest.
- Acutely or chronically cardiac-stressed patients after optimization of volume status if no response to dopamine or dobutamine.

Administration

Through central vein.

Adverse Effects

- Ventricular arrhythmias, myocardial ischemia.
- Arrhythmias particularly with myocarditis; hypokalemia and hypoxemia.
- Pulmonary vascular resistance may increase; hence, judicious use in pulmonary arterial hypertension (PAH).

NOREPINEPHRINE

- $\alpha 1$ and $\beta 1$ activity with no $\beta 2$ activity.
- Adrenergic stimulation dose-dependent, but $\alpha 1$ activity dominates over $\beta 1$ at all doses.
- *<0.5 µg/kg/min:* $\alpha 1 = \beta 1$ vasopressor and inotrope.
- *0.5 µg/kg/min:* $\alpha 1 > \beta 1$ dominant vasopressor:
  - At high doses positive inotropic effect not appreciable because of cardiac response to increased afterload.
  - Heart rate may decrease owing to vagal-mediated baroreceptor reflex secondary to increased afterload.

Indication

- Hyperdynamic septic shock with tachycardia, wide pulse pressure, bounding pulses, warm skin and prolonged capillary refill.
- Severe shock with hypotension with optimal intravascular volume status.

Administration

Always through central line.

Adverse Effects

- Tissue and skin necrosis from peripheral venous site infiltration.
- Compromise of splanchnic, GI and renal blood flows.

DOBUTAMINE

- $\beta 1$, $\beta 2$ and $\alpha 1$ agonist activity.
- *2-20 µg/kg/min:* $\beta 1$ essentially and some $\beta 2$ activity.
- Pure inotrope—increased contractility with decreased systemic vascular resistance (SVR) owing to $\beta 2$ vasodilatory effect.
- *>20 µg/kg/min:* $\beta 1$ and $\alpha 1$ but $\alpha 1$ dominates.

Indications

- Low cardiac output after cardiac surgery with normal or high vascular resistance.
- Myocarditis and dilated cardiomyopathy.

Administration
Through a peripheral or central line.

Adverse Effects
- Less chronotropic and less arrhythmogenic.
- Less tissue necrosis from local infiltration.
- May increase intrapulmonary shunting due to pulmonary vasodilation.

ISOPROTERENOL
- Potent B agonist activity, no α activity; $\beta 1 = \beta 2$ positive inotrope and peripheral vasodilator.
- Also bronchodilator.
- β-agonist, increases with increase in dosage.
- *Starting dose:* 0.05–1.5 µg/kg/minute, and dose increased by 0.05–0.1 µg/kg/minute for every 10–15 minutes until desired effect.
- If heart rate exceeds 200 beats/minute or diastolic pressure falls to <40 mm Hg, dose should not be increased.
- Increases myocardial contractility, heart rate and conduction velocity, and decreases AV Nodal conduction owing to $\beta 1$ agonist activity.
- $\beta 2$ agonist action causes peripheral vascular dilatation, causing reflex tachycardia.
- Cardiac output increases more due to tachycardia than contractility.

Indications
Increase in heart rate in bradycardia from AV block or sinus node dysfunction.

Administration
- Safe through peripheral line.
- *0.1–5.0 µg/kg/min:* $\beta 1 = \beta 2$.

Adverse Effects
Extreme tachycardia, tachyarrhythmia, increased intrapulmonary shunting due to pulmonary vasodilatation.

BIPYRIDINES (PHOSPHODIESTERASE INHIBITORS)
Amrinone
- Inotrope and vasodilator—inodilator.
- 0.75–4.0 µg/kg loading dose used as adjuncts to catecholamines, long half-life.
- *Infants and children:* 5–8 hours.

- 5–20 µg/kg/minute.
- Bolus should be given over 10 minutes, as rapid infusion can cause hypotension from vasodilatation. Bolus to be avoided unless amrinone started on CPB.

Milrinone

- More potent than amrinone.
- 0.5–1 µg/kg/minute; shorter half-life: 30–60 minutes.

Indications

- Useful in patients with β receptor down-regulation [chronic congestive cardiac failure (CCF), chronic stress, septic shock hypodynamic with increased SVR].
- Useful following cardiac surgery [avoid bolus unless milrinone started on cardiopulmonary bypass (CPB)].

Adverse Effects

- Amrinone—thrombocytopenia.
- Milrinone, thrombocytopenia less common, arrhythmias more common.

VASODILATORS

Useful in low cardiac output: Venous and arterial dilatation.

Nitroprusside

- Arterial and venous vasodilatation.
- 0.5–5 µg/kg/minute infusion progressively increased and titrated to desired effect; if BP is still elevated consider other antihypertensives:
  - Thiocyanate and cyanide toxicity in hepatic and renal insufficiency.
  - Rapid action; preload and afterload both decreased.

Indications

Cardiogenic shock, peripheral vasoconstriction, severe systemic hypertension, PAH.

Administration

- Delivery systems and tubing to be protected from light.
- Potentially severe hypotension can be corrected by decreasing rate or cessation of infusion because of short half-life.
- Slow titration of infusion rate with volume optimization.

- Careful use in increased intracranial pressure (ICP) as it may worsen ICP.

Nitroglycerine

- Sublingual, transdermal or IV—0.5-20 µg/kg/min.
- Venous dilation and some arterial dilation at high doses.
- Central venous pressure (CVP), pulmonary capillary wedge pressure (PCWP) and pulmonary artery pressure (PAP) decreased.

Indications
Increased preload with systemic and pulmonary venous congestion in postoperative patients with low cardiac output, CCF and PAH.

Adverse Effects
- Hypotension
- Headache.

Phenoxybenzamine

- *Dose:* 1 mg/kg loading dose in OT, then 0.5 mg/kg/8 hours in PICU.
- Long half-life, noncompetitive alpha-blocker.
- Dosing is by intermittent bolus/infusions for every 8-12 hours.
- Can override by titrating noradrenaline for effect.

Prostacyclin (Epoprostenol)

- *Dose range:* 5-25 µg/kg/min (0.005-0.025 µg/kg/min).
- Profound systemic and pulmonary vasodilator.
- Very expensive, limited availability.
- Antiplatelet action.

VASOCONSTRICTOR

Vasopressin

- Vasopressin is also termed antidiuretic hormone or arginine vasopressin.
- Vasopressin is released in response to a decrease in blood volume or an increase in osmolarity.
- End organ effects are mediated by two receptor subtypes:
  - V1 receptor on vascular smooth muscle cells throughout body causing vasoconstriction.
  - V2 receptors in distal and collecting tubules of the glomeruli and promoting water reabsorption.
  - V3 receptor at posterior lobe of the pituitary gland.
  - V1 effect > V2 effect.

Dose
- In vasodilatory shock after CPB—0.01–0.1 U/min.
- Vasopressin can be diluted to a concentration of 100–1000 U/L in 5% dextrose or NS:
  - *Normal infusion mixture:* 100 U/250 mL.
  - *Dose:* 0.0003 IU/kg/min.
  - *Available strength:* 1 mL = 20 IU.
  - *Dilution:* 20 IU in 40 mL NS.

  1 mL = 0.5 IU

$$CC/HR = \frac{0.0003 \text{ IU} \times \text{weight} \times 60}{20/40}$$

Adverse Effects
- Myocardial ischemia, bronchoconstriction, tremor, facial pallor, vertigo, abdominal cramps.
- Gastric infarction, nausea, vomiting.

LEVOSIMENDAN (INODILATOR)

- Available preparation.
- 12.5 mg per vial as a yellow amorphous powder.
- To be reconstituted only with dextrose (5%) containing solution.

Mechanism of Action
- Calcium sensitizer (pyridazone dinitrile derivative).
- Binds to cardiac troponin C and stabilizes troponin C.
- Triple mode of action—inotropy, vasodilatation and cardioprotection.

Indication
- Low cardiac output syndrome (LCOS).
- Heart failure.

Dosage
- Loading —>6–12 µg/kg over 10 minutes (SBP should be >90 mm Hg).
- Maintenance —>0.05–0.2 µg/kg/min through a central line for 24–48 hours.
- Active metabolite has long t1/2 (75–80 hrs).

Adverse Effects
- Hypotension
- Arrhythmia
- Hypokalemia.

Table 18.1 summarises all inotropes.

TABLE 18.1: Comparison of inotropes.

Clinical effect	Ideal agent	Ionodilators		
		Dobutamine	PDE inhibitor	Levosimendan
COP	↑↑	↑↑	↑↑	↑↑
HR	↔	↑↑	↑	↑/↔
BP	↓	↑	↓↓↓	↓
O_2 demand	↓	↑↑	↑	↔
Arrhythmia potential	↓	↑↑	↑↑	↔
Filling pressure	↓	↓	↓	↓

Chapter 19

Postoperative Anticoagulation

Prashant Shah

INDICATION

- Aortopulmonary shunts:
  - BT shunt
  - Central shunt.
- Cavopulmonary shunts:
  - Bidirectional Glenn procedure
  - Fontan procedure.
- Valve repair or replacement with prosthetic value or ring.
- Atrial fibrillation.
- Systemic emboli.
- Device closure of defects like atrial septal defect (ASD), ventricular septal defect (VSD), patent ductus arteriosis (PDA).

AGENTS USED

- *Aspirine:* Indicated for shunt procedure and cavopulmonary shunts.
  Dose: 2–5 mg/kg/daily along with antacids.
- *Dipyridamole:* 1–2 mg/kg/dose (maximum 100 mg) 6–8 hourly orally.

WARFARIN

- Prosthetic valve replacement.
- Extracardiac fontan procedure.
- Atrial fibrillation.

Dose

- 0.2 mg/kg stat (maximum 10 mg).
- Next day check INR value and if INR <1.3 then increase by 0.05–0.2 mg/kg daily orally.
- Adjust does with INR value.
- Target INR value 2–2.5 for prophylaxis and 2.5–3.5 for prosthetic valve.
- Drug interaction should be considered.

Injection Heparine
- 5–10 IU/kg/hr as a infusion or 50–100 IU/kg/every 6 hourly postoperatively.
- Should start after checking activated partial thromboplastintime (APTT) and activated clothing time (ACT).
- Target APTT/ACT should be 1.5 times then normal.
- Wean heparine once INR reach at target value.

Chapter 20

Routine General Care

K Mahalaxmi, R Kokila

ORAL HYGIENE

Maintained by the nurse-in-charge of the patient:
- Contents of mouth wash bowl:
  – Gauze pieces.
  – Straight artery forceps.
  – Stainless steel bowl (200 mL).

Procedure
- Teaspoonful of dettol in (chloroxylenol + menthol) is added to about 120–150 mL of sterile water in the bowl.
- Gauze pieces are held by artery forceps as soaked in the above solution.
- The teeth are brushed thoroughly and the tongue is mopped.
- This is done every morning.

BLADDER CARE
- All patients routinely catheterized with indwelling (Foley's) catheters prior to surgery.
- Hourly urine output is measured and charted.
- In cases suspected to have a blocked catheter, a bladder wash is performed with sterile water under strict aseptic conditions.
- The catheter is changed if bladder wash is not successful.

BOWEL CARE
- In general all patients kept nil per os (NPO) for 6–8 hours following arrival in the ICU postoperatively. Prolonged NPO for specific cases as advised by the cardiac surgeon.
- Passage of flatus and stools recorded.
- Nasogastric or oral feeds started only after confirming presence of bowel sounds.
- Glycerin suppositories used if patient does not pass stools for >48 hours.

NASOGASTRIC TUBE AND GASTRIC ASPIRATION

- *Sizes available in PICU:* 8F, 10F, 12F, 14F, 16F.
- *Lengths to be inserted:* Distance from the angle of the mouth to the tragus of the ipsilateral ear and then up to the xiphoid process is marked and the tube inserted up to the length measured.
- Injecting air and simultaneous auscultation at gastric area confirms its proper position.

CARE OF URINARY CATHETER

- *Insertion:* Scrubbed well and appropriately sized disposable sterile gloves worn.
- Genitals painted liberally with antiseptic solution (betadine).
- Distal fragment of catheter smeared with xylocaine jelly and catheter inserted perurethra into the bladder.
- The region is cleaned with betadine daily and sterile gauze with betadine ointment is placed at the side in males.
- The catheter is changed every seventh day.
- Culture for microbiology should always be done from the removed catheter tip.

TEMPERATURE

- It is measured by a rectal probe/catheter with a monitor or skin probe.
- Rectal thermometers are not used.
- Common measures used to increase the body temperature if child is cold:
  - Hemotherm—a sheath (having water) is placed beneath the patient and is connected to a machine having different temperature regulator settings.
  - Focusing lamp.
  - Overhead infant radiant warmer for neonates and infants.
- Measures to decrease the body temperature if child is having hyperthermia:
  - Sponging with lukewarm water.
  - Antipyretics—paracetamol parenteral/oral.
  - Hemotherm.

PROTOCOL FOR HYPERTHERMIA

Indication
Hyperthermia exists if rectal temperature is ≥38.3°C (≥101°F).

Rationale

Hyperthermia increases metabolic demands and, thus, myocardial oxygen consumption. Severe hyperthermia [central temperatures ≥41.1°C (≥106°F)] may permanently and severely damage the brain.

Treatment

- If rectal temperature is ≥38.3°C (≥101°F), give acetaminophen as a rectal suppository every 4 hours. The dose in infants and children is 10 mg/kg (rounded to the nearest 30 mg and, in adults, 650–1000 mg).
- Consider using a cooling blanket or cold syringing and a fan or ice bags applied to the body.
- If rectal temperature is ≥39.4°C (≥103°F):
  - Insert esophageal temperature probe for continuous monitoring of central temperature and intensity efforts to improve cardiac output. Check for possible transfusion reaction.
  - If esophageal temperature is ≥39.4°C (≥103°F):
    - Make preparations for peritoneal dialysis with room temperature or cooled dialysate, to be initiated if simpler measures do not promptly control hyperthermia.
    - Give acetaminophen as in step 1.
    - Give dexamethasone, 0.25 mg/kg IV, then 0.1 mg/kg IV every 6 hours.
- Abolish muscular heat production, particularly when an infant is restless, by paralyzing with pancuronium (0.1 mg/kg).
- Continue efforts to improve cardiac output.
- Cold PD cycles (last measure).

ROUTINE CARE OF ORAL OR NASAL ENDOTRACHEAL TUBE

- Ensure patency by regular gentle suctioning every second hour; avoid high-pressure junction.
- Change endotracheal (ET) tube every 7 days.
- Check on proper positioning of the tube in X-rays daily.
- Check for kinking/block of the tube.
- Minimize dead space by short segmenting from the opening of the mouth/nostril.
- Small air leak around the tube is preferred to avoid barotraumas.
- Perform gentle deep suctioning by inserting the suction catheter to about three-fourth of the length of the ET tube.
- Disconnect from ventilator only for a brief period for suctioning.

- Before extubation, check for air leak and, if no air leak, initiate dexamethasone therapy.
- Incidences that may cause disasters:
  - ET tube disconnected from ventilator.
  - ET tube kinking.
  - Block in ET tube owing to mucous or clots.
  - Self-extubation or accidental pullout.

CARE OF EYES

- To avoid exposure keratitis during mechanical ventilation and infant in radiant warmer, use moisol/gel.
- Cover eyes with sterile gauze with eyelids closed.
- Check pupils regularly for size, equality and response to light.
- Fundoscopy for retinal bleed if prothrombin time (PT), activated partial thromboplastin time (APTT) are prolonged or in suspected bleeding disorders and systemic candidiasis.
- On suspicion of keratitis give normal saline wash for every 2 hours.
- In suspected infection, administer local antibiotic therapy (eye drops/ointment).

SKIN CARE

- Nursing care of skin with constant monitoring is vital to prevent skin breakdown.
- Skin should be kept clean and dry.
- Regular turning from one side to other to relieve pressure areas with soft pillows or blanket rolls should be done.
- If patient is immobilized for longer period of days, physical therapy program to be initiated.

TRACHEOSTOMY CARE

- Tracheostomy patient requires the support and individual attention of each member of the care-giving team—doctor, respiratory therapist, nurse, speech therapist and dietician. Tracheostomy is an artificial opening (stoma) made over the neck surface into the windpipe (trachea). A tube is placed through this opening that guards the track. It accomplishes easy passage of air to the lungs, bypassing the naso/oropharyngolaryngeal dead space. The normal naso-oral mucosa and the nasal turbinates function by way of filtering, warming and humidifying the inhaled air. But a tracheostomy patient gets deprived of these functions due to the bypassing. Care of the tracheostomy tube incorporates these basic functions of the bypassed airway.

- *Care of tracheostomy tube:*
    - Humidification—allowance of extra water intake to make up for the insensible water loss through exposed tracheal mucosa, "saline bullets," humidifier or a humidifying machine is used to keep the air humidified for the patient.
    - Stoma care—skin around the opening of the tracheostomy tube needs routine cleaning. This helps prevent skin irritation and any inspissation of secretions and crust formation. Gentle cleaning is accomplished with mild soap water, and any crust is removed with use of diluted hydrogen peroxide (1:1 with water). Mucus sludge is removed with a gauze broth, and finally the tracheostomy ties are adjusted to snuggly fit the tube in place after ruling out any redness or irritation of the stoma skin.
- Precut or handmade tracheostomy gauze dressings are used for the dressing of the stoma skin.
- Suctioning—it is needed to remove mucus or secretions from the airway. Frequency of suctioning needs to be individualized as per the patient needs. Care should be taken not to exceed the diameter of the suction tube to more than half the diameter of the tracheostomy tube. Suction procedure should be aseptic/clean technique. Adequate care needs to be taken to avoid mucosal tears during suctioning.
- *Care of the inner tube:* When using an assembly with an inner tube, it needs a change as per the material, whether disposable or a reusable type, as per the specifications.
- Tracheostomy ties—T will ties or Velcro ties are described for use in practice for securing the tracheostomy tube in place. Always a new tie must be secured prior to removing the old ties. At least a finger should pass between the tie and skin snuggly as to have a secure tie in place.
- Cuffed tracheostomy tube—cuffed tubes are used when ventilating the patient on a ventilator/breathing machine.
- Air filled/water filled or foam cuffs are available.
- Cuffed tracheostomy tubes are available from size 5.5 Fr upward. It helps prevent aspiration of the oronasal as well as stomach contents. Appropriate volume of inflation of cuff achieves a sealed airway and hard proof against any aspirations.
- Overinflation can cause pressure necrosis of the tracheal wall.
- Before the cuff is deflated, it needs to be suctioned before removal to aspirate all the mucus secretions pooled around the cuff seal.

- Changing outer tube (tracheostomy tube)—needs to be done as a hospital policy or as decided by the surgeon/intensivist.
- Fenestrated tracheostomy tube—its use has been to allow patient to have his own breathing through his own nose/mouth. It is also used while weaning from the tracheostomy tube.
- It can also be capped for normal oral and nasal breathing and speaking.

PHYSIOTHERAPY AND ENDOTRACHEAL (ET) SUCTION

- Maintenance of a clear, patent tracheobronchial tree for good air entry during respiration, assisted or spontaneous, is essential.
- Atelectasis from bronchial secretions must receive attention.
- Physiotherapy by percussion, vibration from vibrator and regular gentle suctioning of the ET tube are key to proper management.
- A hand cuplike figure should be made or a silicon cuff should be used for percussion for vibration (Figs. 20.1A and B).

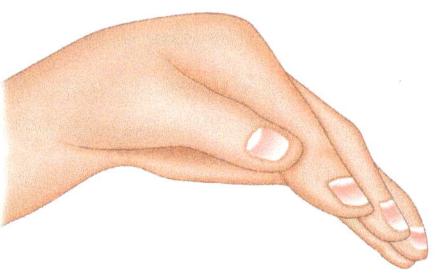

Fig. 20.1A: Position of hand-cuff.

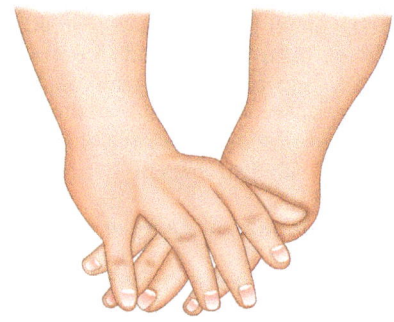

Fig. 20.1B: Position of hand for vibration.

- Mechanical vibrators are of good help for mobilizing of secretions:
  - Once child is extubated, he/she should be encouraged to cough and spit.
  - Deep breathing exercises by blowing balloons should be encouraged.
  - Postural drainage may be required based on region of atelectasis (Fig. 20.2).
  - *Postural drainage:* Patient assuming various positions to facilitate the flow of secretions from various parts of the lung into the bronchi, trachea and throat so that they can be cleared and expelled from the lungs more easily.

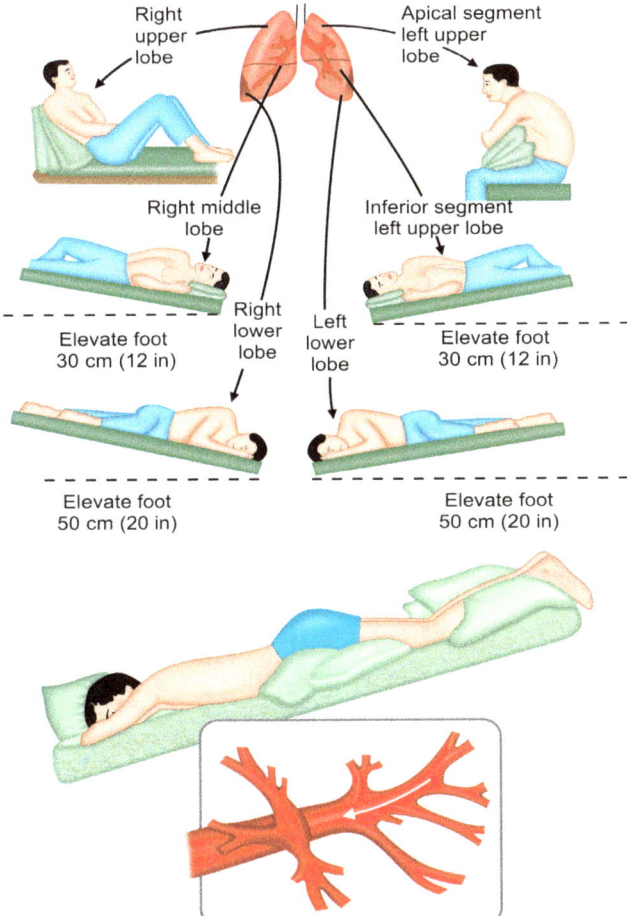

Fig. 20.2: Different positions for postural drainage.

- Physiotherapy in the presence of motor paralysis of limbs from neurological complication should be carried out in consultation with the neurologist.

ENDOTRACHEAL SUCTIONING

- Endotracheal suctioning (ETS) is a necessary practice carried out in the intensive care unit.
- It involves the removal of pulmonary secretion from a patient with an artificial airway in place.
- Make an informed choice about the frequency with which ETS is performed.

Indication

- Decrease in S_aO_2.
- Increase in $ETCO_2$.
- Deterioration in blood gas.
- Increase in the work of breathing, increase in respiratory rate.
- Increase in airway pressure.
- Change in heart rate.
- Atelectasis.

Hazards of Endotracheal Suction

- Arrhythmias.
- Hypoxia.
- Hypo/hypertension.
- Raised intracranial pressure.
- Pulmonary hemorrhage.
- Laryngospasm.
- Infection.
- Staff should constantly be aware of hazards of ETS and should be skilled in the assessment of respiratory function and management of airway.

PREPARING FOR ET SUCTION

- Keep sterile suction bowl, adequate size catheter, Ambu bag, syringe with NS, glove.
- Ask help from other nurse or physiotherapist.
- Sedate patient adequately.
- Disconnect patient from ventilator and hyperventilate with 100% O_2 (for a patient with single ventricle and high pulmonary blood flow, ventilate with room air).
- Carry out suction with adequate suction.
- After suction, hyperventilate for a minimum of 1 minute before connecting back to ventilator.

Size of Suction Catheter
- Size of suction catheter should be large enough to remove secretion effectively and small enough to prevent obstruction.
- The suction catheter should be no more than half the internal diameter of endotracheal tube.

Formula for Selection of Appropriate Suction Catheter
(Size of ETT or tracheostomy tube – 2) × 2 = Size of French catheter.

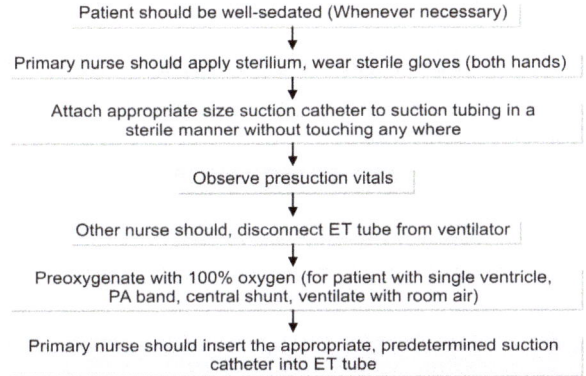

Mobilization of Secretion
- Beside suctioning other methods that make secretion thin and loose helps the removal of secretion.
- Keep secretion thin by:
  - Adequate hydration.
  - Humidification of airway.
  - Using mucolytic agents.
  - Using 2–10 mL of normal saline lavage followed by manual ventilation with bag.

Chapter 21

Infection Issues and Antimicrobials

Prashant Shah, Amit Mishra

INFECTION ISSUES

- Infants and children have a high incidence of nosocomial infections. *Staphylococcus epidermidis, Staphylococcus aureus, Enterococci* and enteric gram-negative bacilli are important pathogens.
- *Diagnosis:* Episodes of fever without evidence of infection is not uncommon. Fever after 48 hours and temperature >39°C should be considered at great risk. Common sites of infection are IV catheters, particularly central lines, respiratory tract, urinary tract and mediastinum.
- Clinical and lab evaluation are vital.
- Regular white blood cell (WBC) counts, C-reactive protein (CRP), erythrocyte sedimentation rate (ESR) and cultures from potential sites (blood tracheal, urinary and wound are appropriate) are diagnostic.

SEPSIS

Fever
- Cardiopulmonary bypass is a potent cause of fever.
- Low cardiac output leads to central hyperthermia and peripheral coolness.

First 24 Hours
- Stress response to cardiopulmonary bypass (CPB).
- Sepsis less common.
- Malignant hyperpyrexia (rare).
- Observation/Paracetamol.
- Rigorous antipyretic measures if fever >38.5°C with poor perfusion or arrhythmia (cooling blanket).

After First 24 Hours
- Low cardiac output.
- Vasodilatation.
- Requiring more cardiovascular support than expected.

Search for Signs
- Lower respiratory tract infection (LRTI)—CXR changes, endotracheal (ET) tube aspiration.
- Otitis media—look in ears.
- Sinusitis—long-term intubated, purulent nasal discharge.
- Septic workup [full blood count (FBC), blood film, blood culture of all central venous catheter (CVC) lumens].
- History of preoperative signs in postoperative patient—usually community acquired/viral.

Hospital-acquired Lower Respiratory Tract Infection
- Moraxella may be associated with flucloxacillin prophylaxis.
- *Haemophilus influenzae*.
- Gram-negatives—coliforms/*Pseudomonas/Enterobacter*.
- Yeasts.
- Treat if systemically unwell or hemodynamically compromised.

Line-related Sepsis
- Primary bacteremia associated with intravascular device may occur.
- Coagulase negative staphylococci is most common.
- Lines should be removed as soon as they are no longer required and if there is a suggestion that they are infected.

PREVENTION
- Wash hands before and after every patient contact.
- Only use patient's allocated stethoscope.
- Replace peripheral IV cannula if inflamed.
- Follow full sterile technique for CVC insertion and handling:
    - Culture all lumens (and tip of CVC if removed) + peripheral site if sepsis suspected.
    - Preferably replace CVC, do not rewire.
    - Treat if systemically unwell or hemodynamically compromised.
- Every PICU must have own "infection protocol," which should be periodically evaluated, modified, if needed, particularly with regard to antimicrobial therapy, both for prophylaxis and curative. The challenging problem of bacterial resistance deserves constant attention.

ANTIBIOTICS
Kindly refer Appendix 1 for all antibiotic doses.

Features of First-, Second-, Third-, Fourth-generation Cephalosporin

First Generation (p Ceph 1): Cephalothin, Cefazolin, Cephapirin, Cephradine, and Cefadroxil

- Most active in comparison to gram-positive cocci. Enterococci are resistant. Limited activity in comparison to aerobic gram-negative bacilli, *E. coli, K. pneumoniae, P. mirabilis.*

Second Generation

- Cefuroxime subgroup (P Ceph 2)—cefuroxime, cefonicid, cofactor, cefuroxime axetil, cefprozil.
- About equal to first-generation cephalosporins in comparison to gram-positive cocci.
- More active in comparison to *E. coli, K. pneumoniae, P. mirabilis.*
- Also active in comparison to β-lactamase positive *H. influenzae, M. catarrhalis*, and relatively resistant (MIC <2 µg/mL) *S. pneumoniae.*
- Cephamycin subgroup (P Ceph 2)—cefoxitin, cefotetan, cefmetazole: Less active than first generation in comparison to gram-positive anaerobes. They are most active in comparison to *Bacteroides* species.

Note: Cefotetan and cefmetazole are less active than cefoxitin in comparison to gram-negative anaerobes other than *B. fragilis.*

Third Generation

- Enhanced activity in comparison to aerobic gram-negative bacilli (P Ceph 3)—cefotaxime. Moxalactam first generation in comparison to gram-positive cocci.
- Most active in comparison to *E. coil, Klebsiella* species, *Proteus* species. Inconsistent in comparison to *Serratia, Enterobacter, Acinetobacter* and *Pseudomonas.*
- Only modest activity in comparison to anaerobes (ceftizoxime most active of the group).
- Enhanced antipseudomonal activity (P Ceph 3 AP)—cefoperazone, ceftazidime: Least active in comparison to aerobic gram-positive cocci. Similar to P Ceph 3 in comparison to aerobic gram-negative bacilli. Most active in comparison to *P. aeruginosa.*

Fourth Generation (P Ceph 4): Cefepime

- Activity in comparison to gram-positive cocci > P Ceph 3.
- Less activity over P Ceph 3 in comparison to enterobacteria and *P. aeruginosa.*

RECOMMENDED ANTIMICROBIAL AGENTS AGAINST SELECTED ORGANISMS

Antimicrobial Agent

Bacterial species	Recommended	Alternative
Bacteroides fragilis species	Metronidazole	Clindamycin
Bordetella pertussis	Erythromycin	TMS/SMX
Brucella species	Doxycycline + either Gentamicin or Rifampin	Doxycycline, TMP/SMX, chloramphenicol
Campylobacter	jejuni Erythromycin	FQ
Chlamydia pneumoniae	Doxycycline	Erythromycin
Chlamydia trachomatis	Doxycycline or Azithromycin	Erythromycin or Ofloxacin
Citrobacter diversus (koseri) C. freundii	IMP or MER	FQ
Clostridium difficile	Metronidazole (po)	Vancomycin (po)
Clostridium tetani	Metronidazole or Pen G	Doxycycline
Enterobacter species (aerogenes, cloacae)	IMP or MER or AP Pen + APAG	TC/CL or PIP/TZ or Ciprofloxacin
Enterococcus faecalis	Penicillin G (Ampicillin) Add Gentamicin for endocarditis or meningitis	Vancomycin Add Gentamicin for endocarditis or meningitis
Enterococcus faecium	β-lactamase, high-level aminoglycoside resist, vancomycin resist	No regimer of proven efficacy. Consultation recommended if patient has endocarditis or other life-threatening infection
Escherichia coli	Sensitive to BL/BLI, cephalosporins, fQ, TMP/SMX, APAG, nitrofurantoin, IMP	Selection of drug depends on site of infection, i.e. UTI. Multiple (po) agents; meningitis P Ceph 3 or MER
Bacterial species	Recommended	Alternative

Contd...

Contd...

Bacterial species	Recommended	Alternative
Haemophilus influenzae (Meningitis, epiglottitis and other life-threatening illness)	Cefotaxime, TMP/SMX, IMP, MER Ceftriaxone, Ciprofloxacin, Ampicillin (if β-lactamase negative), Azithromycin	
Klebsiella pneumoniae	P Ceph 3, FQ, APAG, TC/CL, AM/SB, PIP/TZ	
Legionella species	Erythromycin ± Rifampin	Azithromycin, Clarithromycin, Pefloxacin, Ciprofloxacin, Ofloxacin
Leptospira interrogans	Penicillin G or Doxycycline	
Listeria monocytogenes	Ampicillin	TMP/SMX
Mycoplasma	Erythromycin	Doxycycline
Pneumonia	Azithromycin, Clarithromycin, Dithromycin	
Neisseria meningitidis (Meningococcus)	Penicillin G	Ceftriaxone
Proteus mirabilis (indole −)	Ampicillin	TMP/ZMX
Proteus vulgaris (indole +)	P Ceph 3 or FQ	APAG
Pseudomonas aeruginosa	AP Pen, P Ceph 3 AP, IMP, Tobramycin	Ciprofloxacin, P, Ceph 4 TC/CL, Aztreonam
Salmonella typhi	FQ, Ceftriaxone	Chloramphenicol, Amoxicillin, TMP/SMX
Serratia marcescens	P Ceph 3, IMP, MER, FQ	Aztreonam, Gentamicin
Shigella species	FQ	TMP/SMX and ampicillin resistance (common in Middle East, Latin America)
Bacterial species	Recommended	Alternative
Staphylococcus aureus, methicillin-resistant	Vancomycin	Teicoplanin, linezolid

Contd...

Infection Issues and Antimicrobials

Contd...

Bacterial species	Recommended	Alternative
S. epidermidis	Vancomycin	Vancomycin = Rifampin
Streptococcus Anaerobic (Peptostreptococcus)	Penicillin G	Clindamycin
Streptococcus pneumoniae	Penicillin G	Multiple agents effective
Penicillin–resistant (MIC >2.0)	Vancomycin	P Ceph 3, 4 IMP
Streptococcus pyogenes (Group A, B, C, G, F Streptococcus milleri)	Penicillin G or V	All B lactams, Erythromycin
Yersinia enterocolitica	TMP/SMX or FQ	P Ceph 3 or APAG

[TMP/SMX: trimethoprim/sulfamethoxazole; AP Pen: antipseudomonal penicillin; P Ceph: parental cephalosporins; PRSP: penicillinase-resistant synthetic penicillins; APAG: antipseudomonal aminoglycosides; FQ: fluoroquinolones (ciprofloxacin, ofloxacin, lomefloxacin, enoxacin, pefloxacin) (nor norfloxacin unless specifically indicated); IMP: imipenem + cilastatin; AM/CL: amoxicillin clavulanate; TC/CL: ticarcillin clavulanate; AM/SB: ampicillin sulbactam; Ceftaz: ceftazidime; PIP/TZ: piperacillin-tazobactam; MER: meropenem; BL/BLI: B lactam/B-lactamase inhibitor (AM/CL, TC/CL, AM/SB, or PIP/TZ)].

Chapter 22

Postpericardiotomy Syndrome

Prashant Shah

INTRODUCTION

Postpericardiotomy syndrome (PPS) is an inflammatory febrile condition secondary to reaction involving the pleura and pericardium. Postcardiac surgery is the most common cause, it can however happen after myocardial infarction (Dressler's syndrome), or even rarely following stent or pacemaker lead implantation, blunt or penetrating trauma involving the pericardium.

The incidence is reported to be varying between 2–3% following cardiac surgery. The precise etiology is not known, it is postulated to be an autoimmune response secondary to exposure to antigens after the pericardium is opened. A viral etiology has been proposed but not conclusively proven.

Clinical presentation is usually in the form of low-grade fever, pericardial or pleuritic pain and mild pericardial and pleural effusions developing 1–6 weeks following surgery involving pericardiotomy, which is self-limited resolving over a period of 2–3 weeks.

The temperature is usually around 38–39°C occasionally going up to 40. They usually do not appear ill. Malaise, irritability and decreased appetite are usually associated. Some degree of dyspnea or arthralgias can be complained as well. Vomiting can sometimes be an symptom of impending tamponade particularly in children.

Some patients can have splinting of the chest secondary to pain leading the hypoxemia and retained secretions, which need to be addressed. Pericardial constriction occurs is less than 0.5% of patients and its causal relation with postpericardiotomy syndrome is not conclusively proven.

This condition can progress into early or late cardiac tamponade or even recurrent cardiac tamponade in less than 1% of patients. Recurrences following tapering of anti-inflammatory medication can occur in 10–15% of the patients. Most recurrences occur within the first 6 months of the surgery.

Mediastinitis can also present as fever in the first weeks and its signs can be masked by anti-inflammatory medications given for postpericardiotomy syndrome. The patients should also be carefully examined for any wound discharge or sternal instability before and even after treatment for PPS.

LAB INVESTIGATIONS

- Leukocytosis, elevated ESR and CRP levels.
- Antiheart antibodies titers are high, but are not commonly done. Cardiac enzymes are not useful for diagnosis.
- ECG may simulate pericarditis with global ST elevation and T-wave inversion. Low QRS amplitude is a manifestation of large pericardial effusion.
- Chest radiography my show cardiomegaly with blunting of pleural angles.
- Echocardiography should be obtained in all, initially only small amount of fluid may be seen posterior to left ventricle during systole and is useful in assessing contractility and ruling out evolving tamponade.

TREATMENT

The treatment is anti-inflammatory drugs like aspirin, ibuprofen and naproxen, for a period of 4-6 weeks tapered as the fluid decreases. Patients not responding of NSAIDs may need corticosteroids like prednisone administered for 1 week and tapered over the next 4 weeks.

Corticosteroids can cause rapid resolution of symptoms and is useful in severe or refractory cases.

The role of colchicine in prevention and treatment is not proven. At present no drug is recommended for its prevention.

Recurrent effusions and symptoms have been treated anecdotally with various drugs like immunoglobulins and low dose methotrexate. Patients with significant effusion should have them drained either through subxiphoid approach or catheter guided pericardiocentesis usually left for 24-48 hours while anti-inflammatory medications are started. A pericardial window may be necessary in recurrent cases, opening either into pleural or abdominal cavity.

In summary postpericardiotomy syndrome is a common self-limiting febrile illness following cardiac surgery usually treated with NSAID's for 2-6 weeks. The patients should be carefully followed up for evolving pericardial effusions or any evidence of masked mediastinitis.

Chapter 23

Congenital Heart Defect with Specific Issue

Prashant Shah, Kamlesh Tailor

BLALOCK-TAUSSIG SHUNT (BT SHUNT) (FIG. 23.1)

Systemic to pulmonary shunts are created to establish reliable pulmonary blood flow in patients with reduce pulmonary blood flow. Shunts can be thought of as "artificial arterial ducts" and are typically sited in neonates with, for instance, pulmonary atresia or severe tetralogy of Fallot, who are supported preoperatively by maintaining duct patency with prostaglandin E_1 or E_2 infusions. Shunts are also sited in older infants and children who are not (yet) suitable for complete or definitive cardiac repair.

Preoperatively: Vascular Access

- Try to avoid cannulation of the superior vena cava (SVC) on the side of the proposed shunt as accidental arterial stab/injury may cause hematoma and make proposed surgery difficult or not possible at the most preferred site.

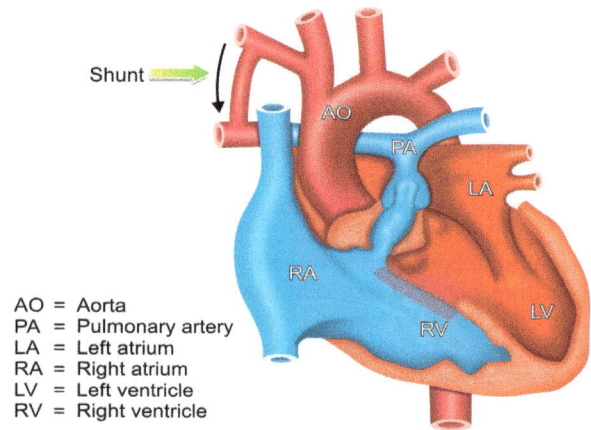

AO = Aorta
PA = Pulmonary artery
LA = Left atrium
RA = Right atrium
LV = Left ventricle
RV = Right ventricle

Fig. 23.1: Blalock-Taussig (BT) shunt.

- Avoid cannulation of the arteries of the shunt side arm as pressure readings will be unreliable both intra- and postoperatively.

Physiology Alteration

After BT shunt surgery quotient of blood flow to pulmonary circuit increases suddenly as compare to preoperative status; and hence, heart work load increases, which causes volume overload to the heart:
- Steal blood from aorta and supply to pulmonary artery.
- Increase blood to same side of lung.
- Regulate flow by size of the graft.

Goal to Manage BT Shunt Patient

- Balancing pulmonary and systemic circulation.
- Optimize the oxygen delivery to tissue.

Postoperative Management

- Maintain adequate cardiac output with use of inotropes—Dopamine or Adrenaline.
- *Adequate hydration:* 80–100 mL/kg/day.
- *Start heparin:* 5–10 units/kg/h.
- *Aspirin:* 5 mg/kg/day.
- Keep FiO_2 as low as possible to achieve target saturation around 70–80%.
- Small children require ventilation for 24 hours—as they tend to go into low cardiac output and same side pulmonary edema.
- Respiratory care—ET toileting, low pressure suction, good chest physiotherapy.

Under-Flowing Shunt: Low Saturations (<65%)

- If the saturation is low (<65%) despite normal BP, normal ventilatory parameters, and clinically normal air entry and chest X-ray (CXR), suspect a malfunctioning shunt (listen for shunt murmur).
- Inform surgeon; obtain an echocardiogram urgently to assess shunt flow.
- Use heparin infusions (10–20 units/kg/h) in situations where shunt occlusion is believed to be a particularly high-risk.
- May need noradrenaline to increase systemic driving pressure in the interim.
- If patient's hematocrit is very high, do phlebotomy and exchange it with saline.

High Flowing Shunt: High Saturations (>85%)
- If shunt flow is excessive the lungs are relatively overperfused and the circulation is unbalanced.
- Suspect excessive shunt if:
  - Saturations exceed 85% at lowest FiO_2.
  - There is pulmonary plethora/edema (may be unilateral).
  - There is cardiac failure.
  - Systemic diastolic pressure is low (due to "run off" through the lungs).
  - There is persistent metabolic acidosis in a "pink" patient (reduced systemic blood flow).

Management of "Over Shunting"
- In relatively modest "over shunting" all that may be needed is restriction of fluid ± diuretics and inotropes (to support the volume-loaded ventricle).
- In more refractory cases, manipulation of pH (permissive hypercapnia) and FiO_2 (lowering) act to raise pulmonary vascular resistance and may assist in reducing pulmonary recirculatory shunt.
- Echocardiography or cardiac catheter may be required to define shunt flow and possible additional sources of pulmonary blood flow such as a patent arterial duct or major aortopulmonary collateral vessels (MAPCAs).
- Urgent surgical revision of a large shunt may occasionally be required (insertion of a smaller diameter shunt). This is certainly the case when very low diastolic pressures and acidosis persist despite medical measures to raise pulmonary vascular resistance.

Seroma
Gortex shunts can "sweat," resulting in a seroma, detected on echocardiography or CXR.

BI-DIRECTIONAL GLENN SHUNT (BDG SHUNT) (FIG. 23.2)
Also known as partial cavopulmonary connection:
- Shunt between SVC and pulmonary artery.
- Indicated for single ventricle physiology with reduced pulmonary blood flow.

Anesthesia Management
- Place short neck line/internal jugular line to measure Glenn pressure postoperatively.

Congenital Heart Defect with Specific Issue

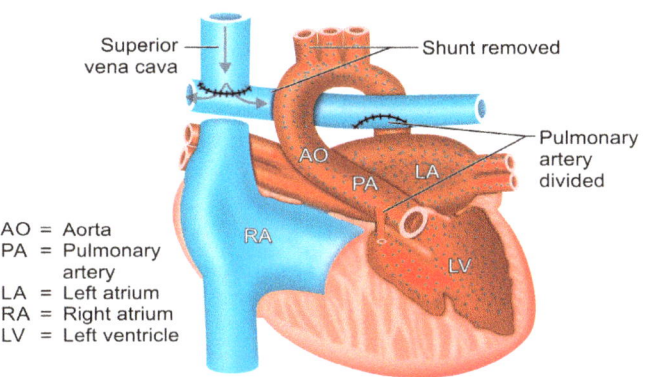

Fig. 23.2: Bidirectional Glenn shunt.

- Femoral line requires to measure ventricular filling pressure.

Postoperative Management

- Head up position, which augments SVC blood to pulmonary circuit.
- Ventilatory settings with lower mean airway pressure and low PEEP.
- Early weaning from ventilator owing to spontaneous ventilation.
- Venous returns to be augmented.
- Negative intrapleural pressure—lowers pulmonary artery pressure—improves Glenn flow to pulmonary arteries.
- Strictly avoid hyperthermia postoperatively as these are very susceptible to brain insult due to compromised cerebral venous drainage. Head cooling advisable for first 12–24 hours postoperatively.
- Hypercarbia and hypoxemia as potential pulmonary vasoconstrictors to be avoided.
- Injection heparin 5–10 units/kg/h to be started after 4 hours.
- Aspirin 5 mg/kg/h on next day—after two doses of tablet aspirin, heparin to be stopped.
- Neckline to be taken out early.
- If child develops facial edema, congestion or irritability, Glenn flow to be checked by echo.
- All single ventricles to be taken care during injection to prevent air embolization.

High-risk BDG

- Patients with high pulmonary artery pressure (mean >18).
- Borderline pulmonary artery size.
- Patients have high Glenn pressure; to be managed with pulmonary vasodilators like milrinone infusion, and oral sildenafil, once ruling out surgical narrowing at the site of anastomosis between SVC—PA.
- Intermittent hyperventilation with 100% O_2 can improve Glenn flow.

PULMONARY ARTERY BANDING (FIG. 23.3)

- An artificial obstruction to pulmonary artery is created to reduce blood flow to PAs in subset where excessive PA flow can cause cardiac failure.
- Indication for PA band.
- Single ventricle with increase pulmonary blood flow.
- Swiss cheese ventricular septum or multiple VSDs in sick child.
- D-TGA intact septum after 3 weeks along with BT shunt to train LV.

Physiology Alteration by Surgery

- Reduced PA flow—low saturation.
- Blood diverted from PAs to aorta, so increase in systemic pressure.
- Increased right ventricular afterload.

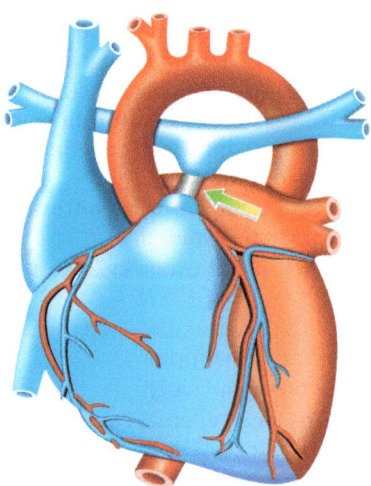

Fig. 23.3: Pulmonary artery band.

- Sometimes, existing A-V valve leak may increase:
  - During surgery assess band at room air, low tidal volume.
  - Adequacy of band—75–80% saturation, no tachycardia, in single ventricle physiology and around 95% saturation in multiple VSD or two ventricle physiology.

Postoperative Management

As vetricular afterload increases, small dose of milrinone with/without adrenaline help the ventricular dysfunction in first 24 hour:
- Avoid early extubation as this child tend to develop low cardiac output within first 24 hours.
- Good respiratory care is important for this group of patients continuous monitoring of heart rate and saturation is mandatory as these patients suddenly go into bradycardia and desaturation.
- Adding captopril may help ventricle if pressure is good on 2 or 3 pod.
- If these patients' SPO_2 is high, it suggests loose band—do echo and tighten the band.
- Aggressive diuretic therapy is required.

FONTAN PROCEDURE (FIG. 23.4)

- Also known as total cavopulmonary connection.
- Procedure entails connection of systemic venous drainage to pulmonary arteries.
- Either directly by PTFE conduit (extracardiac Fontan) or through right atrium (lateral tunnel Fontan).
- The net pulmonary flow is pressure gradient dependent between systemic venous and pulmonary arterial pressure.

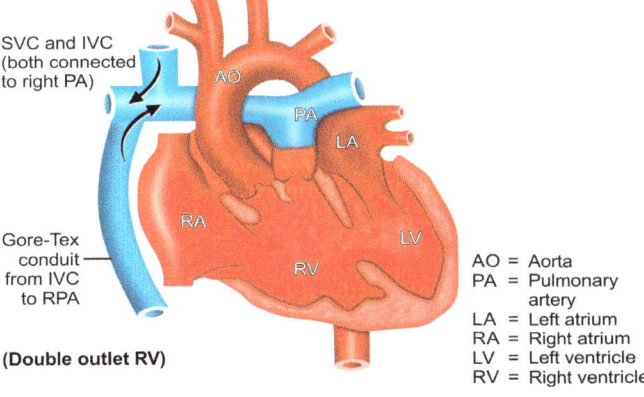

Fig. 23.4: Extracardiac Fontan.

- In high PA pressure or high LA pressure Fontan circuit will not work properly, leads to pleural effusion.
- Fenestration (between Fontan circuit and RA) acts like pop-up valve which reduces venous pressure and improves cardiac output but at the cost of reduction in saturation.

Postoperative Management

- Head up and leg up (Favaloro's) position postoperatively.
- Aim of ventilation strategies will be the same like BDG-less PEEP and early extubation.
- Maintain adequate filling pressure as Fontan circuit flow heavily depend on optimal preload by colloid infusion.
- Good chest physiotherapy is mandatory. It helps for reducing lung atelectasis and hence decreases pulmonary vascular resistant.
- Optimize myocardial contractility, use inodilators.
- In lateral tunnel Fontan, sinus rhythm is mandatory (because it augments cardiac output by 30–50% in a case of single ventricle with Fontan).
- In extracardiac Fontan, start heparin and on extubation, tablet Warfarin; keep INR-2.5–3.
- Watch IVC pressure, which is Fontan pressure; if there is low SPO_2 and high Fontan pressure, do echo immediately to rule out Fontan circuit block.
- Plural effusion is known and may remain for longer time.
- Ascitis may develop in high-risk Fontan.

Special Circumstances

- Owing to sudden reduction of ventricular load change and ventricular geometry change, it goes into ventricular failure, which requires high inotropic support.
- Better to start milrinone along with inotropes.
- Oral sildenafil.
- High FiO_2 if indicated.
- Fenestration will help by decompressing Fontan circuit.
- Despite all measures, if patient's Fontan pressure remain high, do very large fenestration or take down Fontan.

ATRIAL SEPTAL DEFECT (FIG. 23.5)

- This is a acyanotic heart disease with increased pulmonary blood flow.
- These patients have large RA, RV, main pulmonary artery (due to volume overload) and relatively small LA (underfilled).

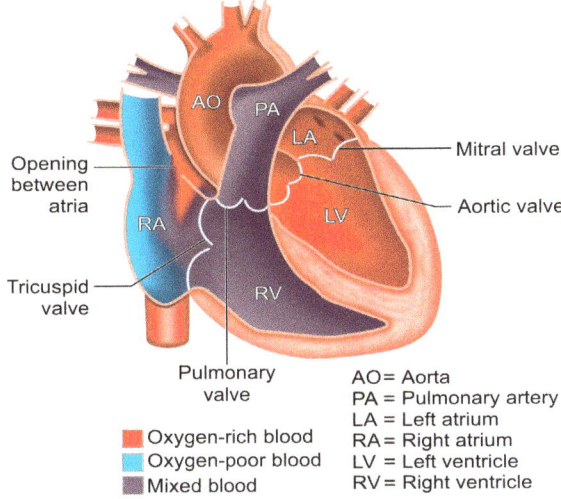

Fig. 23.5: Atrial septal defect (ASD).

Postoperative Management

- Most of these patients have uneventful recovery:
  - Early extubation in operation room or in ICU advisable.
- Avoid infusing large volume boluses; because of small LA may not able to accommodate it and patient can develop pulmonary edema:
  - Small bolus of Lasix before extubation will prevent sudden pulmonary edema in these simple cases.
- Tachypnea, tachycardia and persistent low SPO_2, one should suspect either possibility of pulmonary edema or IVC baffle to LA.
- Arrhythmia of atrial origin may occur.

VENTRICULAR SEPTAL DEFECT (FIG. 23.6)

- Acyanotic heart disease with increase pulmonary blood flow.
- Large LA, LV and main pulmonary artery (due to volume overload).
- Depend on the size of the VSD, the child will have pulmonary hypertension (PAH) from mild to severe.

Postoperative Management

- Early surgical closure advisable in moderate-large VSD to avoid irreversible changes develop in pulmonary vascular bed (Eisenmenger syndrome) due to high pulmonary blood flow.
- Postoperatively, milrinone or dobutamine (inodilator) is the drug of choice in a child with VSD-severe PAH.

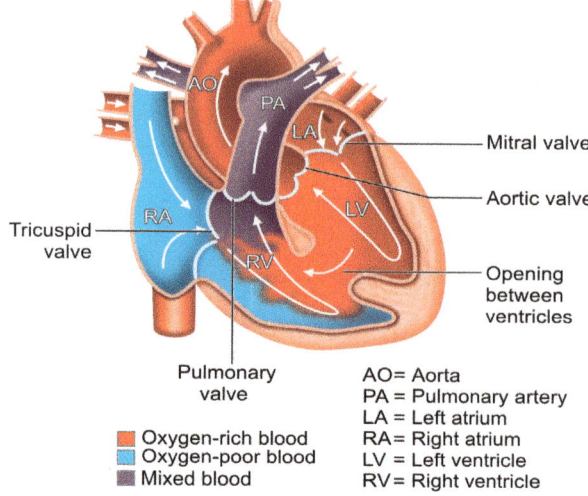

Fig. 23.6: Ventricular septal defect (VSD).

- Early extubation or fast tracking is advisable in a child with small to moderate size VSD.
- Large VSD with severe PAH, the old concept of elective ventilation for next 48 hours is questionable and early extubation within first 24 hours is safe, if child is having stable hemodynamic, normal ABGs, warm periphery and adequate urine output.
- Bolus or continuous infusion of Lasix should be started postoperatively to keep the child negative fluid balance and it will hastened up the extubation process.
- Nutrition supplementation will play important role in treating such patients as most of these patients have low weight/malnutrition because of preoperative congestive heart failure (failure to thrive).

ATRIOVENTRICULAR CANAL DEFECT (FIG. 23.7)

- Acyanotic heart disease with increase pulmonary blood flow.
- Volume overloaded ventricle with severe PAH.
- Early surgical closure is the only treatment to prevent Eisenmenger syndrome.
- Balanced AV canal defect where both the ventricle and AV valve adequate size—biventricular repair is the treatment of choice.
- Unbalanced AV canal defect where one of the ventricle and/or AV valve is small in size—should be treated like single ventricle.

Congenital Heart Defect with Specific Issue

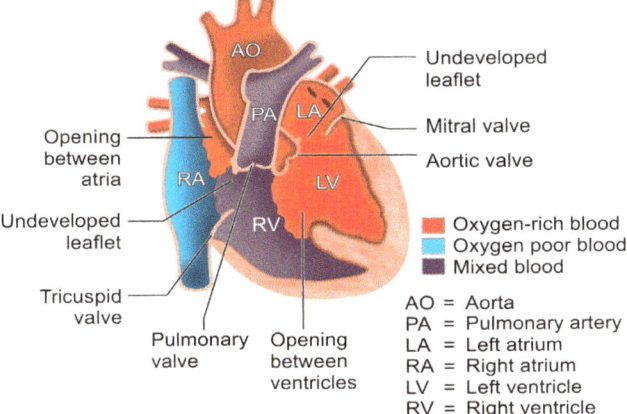

Fig. 23.7: Atrioventricular canal defect (A-VCD).

- Almost 40-50% of AV canal defect patients having associated Down's syndrome.

Postoperative Management

- Inodilator like milrinone is the drug of choice postoperatively with either low dose dopamine or adrenaline.
- Adequate surgical repair of both AV valve is the deciding factor for the smooth course of such patients postoperatively.
- Unable to wean from ventilation or unexplained low cardiac output or severely congested bilateral lung field, one should suspect moderate to severe mitral regurgitation and may require resurgery to correct it.
- Avoid hypertension and excessive child struggling, which may damage surgical AV valve repair.
- Early extubation within first 24 hours of ICU is safe after reconfirming postoperative. Detail echo-check for AV valve regurgitation and ventricular function.
- In case of Down's syndrome, additional sedation may require after extubation and intensivist should be aware/expect some airway problem in such cases.
- Noninvasive ventilation will help in some of case where respiratory efforts are not adequate or lung congestion present.

TOTAL ANOMALOUS PULMONARY VENOUS CONNECTION (TAPVC) (FIG. 23.8)

- Draining of all pulmonary vein into right atrium.
- Three variant—supracardiac, cardiac and infracardiac.
- Obligatory shunt through ASD/PFO from right atrium to left atrium.

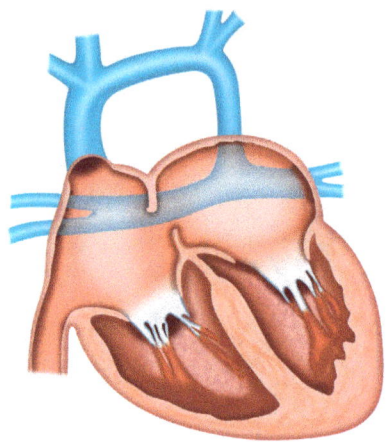

Fig. 23.8: Supracardiac TAPVC.

- Emergency surgery is required if obstruction present at any level of these pulmonary venous drainage.

Postoperative Management

- Management depends upon severity of defect, preoperative PA pressure and status of ventricular function.
- These patients have severe PAH, so management is as follows:
  - Ventilate these patients electively—probably first 24–48 hours.
  - During ventilation keep them heavily sedated.
  - Avoid suction frequently; and if require sedate adequately.
  - Avoid high $PaCO_2$, which can increase pulmonary vascular resistance.
  - If PAH crisis, one should hyperventilate with 100% FiO_2.
  - Milrinone—inotrope of choice with/without Adrenaline as these patients have biventricular dysfunction.
  - Sildenafil intravenous or oral may require if PA pressure remain uncontrolled (rule out respiratory and surgical cause first before starting sildenafil).
  - Keep lungs in a good condition; any atelectasis, pneumothorax, effusion may cause PAH crisis.

TETRALOGY OF FALLOT (FIG. 23.9)

- Cyanotic congenital heart disease.
- The four components of TOF are:
  - VSD

Congenital Heart Defect with Specific Issue

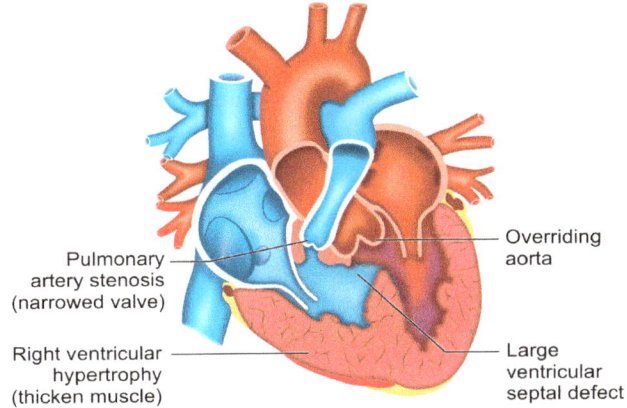

Fig. 23.9: Tetralogy of Fallot.

- Infundibular stenosis
- Overriding of aorta
- Right ventricular hypertrophy.

Before Repair

- Infants with Fallot's have poor tolerance of vasodilators and beta agonists.
- Hypercyanotic spells are usually caused by spasm of right ventricular outflow tract (RVOT) and are treated by:
  - Oxygen.
  - *Volume expansion:* 10–30 mL/kg.
  - Sedation (morphine).
  - Turning infant into knee chest position, where possible.
  - Vasoconstrictor.
  - *Metaraminol:* 0.01 µg/kg stat, then 0.1–1 µg/kg/min.
  - *Noradrenaline infusion:* 0.1–0.5 µg/kg/min.
  - *Beta-blocker—propranolol:* 0.1 mg/kg IV.
  - Intubation/ventilation.

Postoperative Course

- Low cardiac output may result from right ventricular dysfunction due to ventriculotomy, cardiopulmonary bypass (CPB) and residual RVOT obstruction.
- Third spacing is common—require PD or chest tube to drain fluid.
- Maintain a high RA pressure postoperatively to improve cardiac output and also to overcome outflow obstruction.
- Blood or colloid infusion required to improve adequate peripheral perfusion and maintain CVP with colloid.

- RA pressure maintained around 16–18 mm Hg.
- Use inotropes judiciously.

Do not reduce inotropes for 48 hours as they might go into low cardiac output after 12–24 hours:

- Extubation is done with minimal hemodynamic support and FiO_2 of <0.35%.
- Fluid restriction to two-thirds of maintenance.
- Digoxin may be required on weaning from inotropic infusion.
- Right bundle branch block (RBBB) may be caused by ventriculotomy with/without trauma to the right bundle branch or proximal conducting system.
- RBBB is associated with left anterior hemiblock (LAH).
- LAH is associated with complete heart block (CHB).
- Temporary pacing wires are placed during surgery in all patients.
- If CHB persists beyond 2–3 weeks then PPI needed.
- Late complication is ventricular arrhythmias.
- Children with early repair have lesser incidence of ventricular ectopic.
- If patient is in low cardiac output despite high inotropic support, do echo to find out residual VSD, RVOT obstruction, multiple or large AP collaterals and infection.

These patients require good diuretics postoperative; watch liver enlargement and plural effusion, which gives information about RV function.

TRUNCUS ARTERIOSUS (FIG. 23.10)

- Characterized by a single common ventricular outflow tract with a ventricular septal defect.
- Children with good pulmonary blood flow do not require intervention until the PVR falls at the age of 3 months, when significant pulmonary congestion may develop.

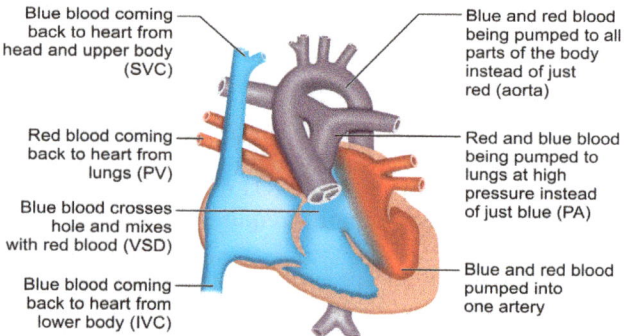

Fig. 23.10: Truncus arteriosus.

- This is high pulmonary blood flow situation so early development of PAH occurs.

Postoperative Care
- Immediate postoperative complications include a decreased cardiac output due to ventriculotomy and PAH.
- All care to prevent PAH crisis as seen early.
- CVP should be increased to maintain cardiac output.
- Fluid is infused at two-thirds maintenance.
- Watch for PAH crisis.
- Infants who do poorly may have truncal valve regurgitation and may require valve repair.
- Cardiac cath and echo to rule out any residual VSD and pulmonary conduit obstruction.

COARCTATION OF AORTA (FIG. 23.11)
- Occurs in descending thoracic aorta, opposite the insertion of the ductus arteriosus and adjacent to the origin of the left subclavian artery.
- Surgical corrections:
  - Subclavian aortoplasty.
  - End-to-end anastomosis.
- Choice is dependent upon the age of the child.
- Intraoperatively during the period of aortic cross clamping, adequacy of perfusion is dependent upon the extent of collateral circulation.
- Ischemia of spinal cord, kidneys and gastrointestinal (GI) tract may result from hypoperfusion.
- Sudden increase in left ventricular afterload may be poorly tolerated by the patient with preexisting CCF.

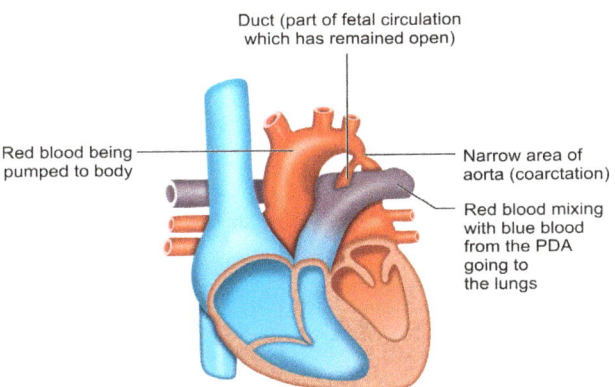

Fig. 23.11: Coarctation of aorta.

- Afterload reduction with vasodilators as nitroprusside can be hazardous with poor distal pressure below the cross clamp.
- Severe complication is paraplegia due to anterior spinal artery syndrome from cross clamping.
- Postoperative atelectasis, even re-expansion of the collapsed left lung from thoracotomy for repair may result.
- Weaning from ventilation and extubation may be delayed due to phrenic nerve and recurrent laryngeal nerve injuries.
- Chylothorax from thoracic duct injury can occur.
- Persistent hypertension is seen after COA repair due to elevated catecholamine and renin levels.
- If untreated, leads to stress on the aortic suture line with excessive bleeding requiring transfusion and even re-exploration.
- Untreated hypertension can lead to postcoarctectomy syndrome—reflex mesenteric vasoconstriction with splanchnic hypoperfusion with resultant intestinal ischemia and perforation causing morbidity and mortality.
- Treatment is NG suction and withholding feed for 2–3 days.
- Nitroprusside, beta-blockers can be used to control hypertension. Captopril: 1–2 mg/kg/dose/8 hours.
- BP should be checked in the legs for presence of any residual gradient.

AORTIC STENOSIS (FIG. 23.12)

- Older patients will be asymptomatic with severe myocardial compromise.
- Etiology is congenital, commonly with bicuspid valve.

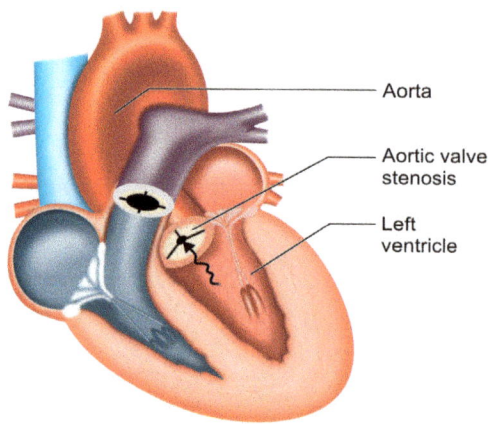

Fig. 23.12: Aortic stenosis.

- Severe aortic stenosis; coronary perfusion is decreased leading to angina and myocardial ischemia.
- Surgical repair is either valvuloplasty or valve replacement.
- Valvuloplasty in infants and valve replacement in the older children.
- Prosthetic valves require life-long coagulation.
- Allografts do not require anticoagulation but tend to deteriorate over time.
- Valvuloplasty may be followed by trivial AR.
- Prosthetic valves may require replacement at a later time.
- Ross procedure consists of replacement of aortic root with native pulmonary valve and replacement of native pulmonic valve with allograft.

Postoperative Management

- Postoperative these patients require high filling pressure, so keep CVP more than 10.
- Extubation should be elective.
- Keep afterload reduction—inodilators.
- Start ACE inhibitors postoperative.
- If prosthetic valve—start injection heparin 10 units/kg/h.
- *Warfarin:* 5 mg/day; maintain INR: 2.5–3.
- *Aspirin:* 5 mg/kg/day.
- *Ross procedure:* Avoid vigorous chest physiotherapy as conduit is lying just below chest cavity.

TRANSPOSITION OF GREAT ARTERIES (FIG. 23.13)

- The surgical procedures currently done are arterial switch (JATENE) or atrial switch (mustard or senning).
- The arterial switch procedure involves reimplanting both great arteries on their respective normal ventricle, with reimplantation of coronary artery into aorta in its new site. This procedure can be done only when the left ventricle can withstand pumping against systemic vascular resistance.
- This occurs under three circumstances:
  - In the few days after birth when the left ventricle had been exposed to high PVR (before 3 weeks).
  - In the presence of a large unrestricted VSD or PDA with high left ventricular pressure and consequently muscle mass in the older child.
  - In the older child with an intact ventricular septum, left ventricular muscle mass is built up over several days by surgically banding the pulmonary artery, allowing the ventricle to hypertrophy and then performing arterial switch.

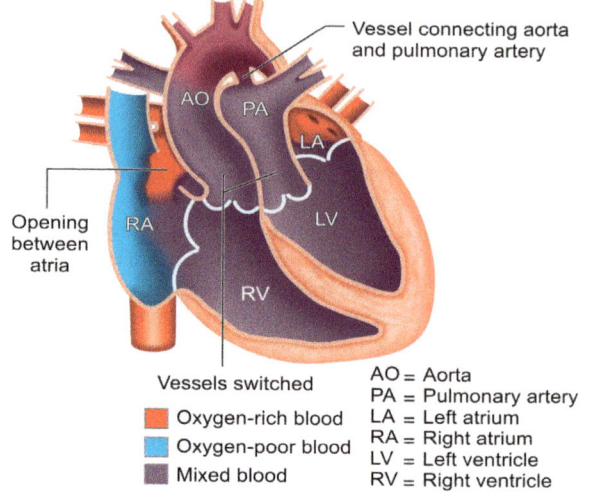

Fig. 23.13: Transposition of great arteries (TGA).

- *Perioperative complications:* Include extensive hemorrhage, elevated PVR and myocardial ischemia related to coronary artery implantation.
- Hemorrhage is multifactorial.
- Large priming volume used in CPB.
- Decreased platelet number and function during bypass and hypothermia.
- The large number and extent of suture lines, which may be in areas not safely accessible.
- Elevated PVR in neonates may lead to right ventricular dysfunction and can be prevented by avoiding hypercarbia and hypoxemia. PAH may require pulmonary vasodilator or inhaled NO.
- Myocardial ischemia can be related to air or other microscopic debris in the coronary arteries.
- Significant embolization can cause overt ventricular failure.
- Coronary artery kinking during the anastomosis also causes ventricular hypoperfusion and ischemia.

Arterial Switch Procedure

Postoperative Care

- Most of the switch babies are neonates and they come to PICU with open chest.
- Nurse open chest patients with extra-aseptic precaution (*see* Appendix 4).

- These patients have LA and PA line; monitor them carefully, keep LAP 10–12, balance it with colloid, fresh frozen plasma (FFP), packed cell volume (PCV).

Restrict fluid up to 800 mL/m^2/day:

- Elective peritoneal dialysis may help to remove extra fluid. Adrenaline, dopamine and milrinone are good inotropic choices.
- Watch for patch bulging and other cardiac tamponade signs—call surgeon.
- Avoid high tidal volume, it may cause tamponade effect and lowers pressure.

Pressure control mode is choice of ventilation:

- Keep all precaution to prevent PAH crisis as described in earlier chapter.
- Maintain heart rate at 140–160; if required, pace atria or atrioventricularly.
- Maintain body temperature by warmer.
- Be vigilant for low cardiac output signs.
- In case of borderline blood pressure, watch for patch bulge.
- Keep adequate filling pressure, if require increase inotropes.
- Keep low threshold for re-exploration.
- If patient remains stable for 24 hours, plan to close the chest.
- During chest closure, watch for change in tidal volume and saturation.
- After chest closure, there is a chance to go into low cardiac output, so step up inotropes if required and start weaning from ventilator once all parameters are acceptable.

ANOMALOUS LEFT CORONARY ARTERY FROM PULMONARY ARTERY (ALCAPA) (FIG. 23.14)

Postoperative management depends upon age of presentation, secondary changes in LV and type of surgery:

- In case of coronary transfer watch for any ECG changes, be alert about kinking of coronary artery or tunnel obstruction.
- Send cardiac enzymes on receipt of patient and repeat after 24 hours.
- Injection milrinone with injection adrenalin is a good choice of inotropes.
- In severe LV dysfunction, intra-aortic balloon pump (IABP) or left ventricle assist device is a good choice in the early postoperative period.

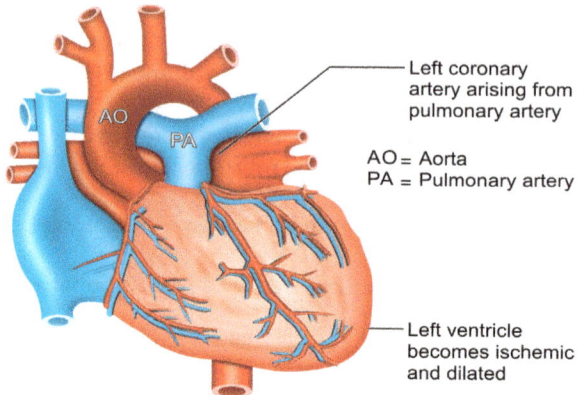

Fig. 23.14: Anomalous left coronary artery from pulmonary artery (ALCAPA).

HYPOPLASTIC LEFT HEART SYNDROME (HLHS)

Early Management

- Hypoplastic left heart syndrome (HLHS) is the most common cardiac malformation causing death from congenital heart disease in the first month of life. The syndrome is a spectrum of left-sided cardiac malformations including aortic atresia or stenosis, hypoplasia of the ascending aortic arch and hypoplasia or absence of the left ventricle. The long-term outlook for babies with this condition was until recently very poor, but two treatment options now offer hope. These options are heart transplantation and staged reconstructive surgery pioneered by Norwood, to reconstruct a viable circulation.
- Neonatal cardiac transplantation is only available in a few centers worldwide; its growth is limited not by any absence of facilities or skill, but by the very limited availability of suitably small donor hearts. The Norwood sequence of operations is therefore the only realistic option for most babies with hypoplastic left heart syndrome (HLHS).
- The first stage of the Norwood sequence aims to reconstruct the aortic arch, ensure adequate mixing with an atrial septectomy and secure pulmonary blood flow with a central or modified Blalock-Taussig shunt or RV-PA conduit (Sano). The aim of the intensivist should be to present babies for this operation with a Qp:Qs as close to 1.0 as possible. Duct patency must be maintained preoperatively with prostaglandin E1 or E2 (*see* below).

- The Stage 1 operation is followed at 4–9 months of age by formation of a bidirectional cavopulmonary connection (Norwood Stage 2), reducing volume load to the ventricle. Finally a "completion" Fontan procedure (Norwood Stage 3) is undertaken, typically at 12–24 months of age.

Presentation

Antenatal Diagnosis

The diagnosis of HLHS is frequently made antenatally on fetal ultrasound screening. Close liaison is then required between the obstetrician, neonatologist and pediatric cardiologist to ensure that the newborn infant is managed appropriately and transferred promptly to a pediatric cardiac unit.

Postnatal Diagnosis

If not diagnosed antenatally, infants with HLHS often present at the time of arterial duct closure with severe shock, acidosis and absent or severely reduced femoral pulses. Their presentation is clinically indistinguishable from severe aortic coarctation. Detailed diagnosis is made by echocardiography following resuscitation.

Echocardiographic Diagnosis

Apart from the basic anatomical arrangement, certain key information is required from the echocardiographer to assist resuscitation. Key points of interest to the intensivist are the status of the arterial duct, and the degree of restriction (if any) to outflow of blood from the left atrium.

A restrictive ASD might be managed by early surgery (best option) or balloon dilation of the ASD (delaying definitive surgery).

Management at Presentation

Survival is determined initially by the following factors:
- Continued ductal patency, ensuring that pulmonary arterial blood reaches the aorta.
- Pulmonary venous return to the left atrium can reach the right heart via patent foramen ovale or ASD.
- A balance is achieved between systemic (SVR) and pulmonary vascular resistances (PVR) such that systemic and pulmonary blood flows are similar ($Qp:Qs \approx 1:1$).
- Prostaglandin infusion to maintain or reopen arterial duct.
- Resuscitation "ABC".
- In antenatally diagnosed cases or when postnatal diagnosis of HLHS is confirmed a number of diagnosis specific management strategies should be implemented.

Airway and Ventilation

- Many babies with HLHS cope well in air (or low FiO_2) on low-dose prostaglandin E1 (PGE1). They are not "automatically" sick and in need of intubation or ventilation.
- If intubation is necessary, limit FiO_2 to 0.21–0.30. Use ketamine + muscle relaxant for "elective" intubations.
- Nurse babies in air or in a head-box in as low as FiO_2 as possible, to maintain systemic arterial oxygen saturations of 70–80%.
- Fully variable blended gas supply should be available for hand ventilation and head-box delivery.
- Do not use nasal oxygen catheters or oxygen masks percentage of delivery is unreliable.
- Initial ventilator setting:
  - *FiO_2:* 0.21–0.30
  - *Rate:* 20/min
  - *TV:* 10 mL/kg.
- Initial blood gas targets:
  - *PaO_2:* 30–45 mm Hg
  - *$PaCO_2$:* 37.5–45 mm Hg
  - *SaO_2:* 70–80% with the aim of optimizing Qp: Qs at 1.

Cardiovascular

- Continue prostaglandin infusion (PGE1 or PGE2 5–20 ng/kg/min).
- Aim for systemic mean arterial pressure 45–60 mm Hg and "good" systemic perfusion (warm peripheries, no base deficit, lactate <2.0).
- Volume expansion using appropriate colloid solutions may be required.
- Consider inotropic support if poor RV function on echo or persisting low output/metabolic acidosis (dopamine 5–15 mg/kg/min), but beware of altering PVR/SVR balance. If dopamine raises PVR then dobutamine may be substituted. Adrenaline remains the universal "second line" agent.

Vascular Access

- These babies are embarking on a surgical course involving at least three major heart operations. All vascular access sites should be treated with great care.
- Multilumen catheters in the SVC should be avoided if at all possible. If SVC sites (IJ or SC) are used, removal should be planned early in the postoperative period.
- However, a single small catheter placed in the SVC is invaluable for monitoring of "mixed venous" oxygen and, therefore, interpreting the balance of shunts in the

period during and immediately after a Norwood Stage 1. Systemic saturations cannot be interpreted adequately without this additional information.
- Left-arm arterial lines should be avoided. HLHS babies often have a coarctation, and at the end of extensive arch repair pressures measured in the left subclavian artery distribution may not be reliable.

BALANCING SHUNTS PREOPERATIVELY

Excessive Pulmonary Blood Flow
- Saturation >80% and PaO_2 >45 mm Hg suggests Qp:Qs >1.
- Low systemic diastolic pressure:
  - Nurse in air.
  - Consider intubation and elective hypoventilation to increase CO_2 to reduce Qp.

Low Pulmonary Blood Flow
- Saturation <70% suggests Qp:Qs <1.
- It is relatively rare before Stage I repair.
- Check prostaglandin delivery:
  - Confirm ductal patency and revisit ASD (restrictive) on echo.
  - Try systemic vasoconstrictor (noradrenaline 0.05–0.4 mg/kg/min) while arranging emergency surgery if saturations do not improve quickly.

Timing of Surgery
- If the baby is relatively stable, the Stage I Norwood procedure should be performed either on the day of admission or the day following admission during daylight hours.
- If the baby is unstable, despite appropriate management and surgery is not contraindicated by major concurrent problems, surgery should be arranged urgently.
- Surgery may occasionally be postponed to facilitate neurological assessment if it is believed that the baby has been so sick at presentation that major neurological handicap is likely.

Surgery and Anesthesia
While styles of anesthesia vary, the following key points apply generally:
- Shunt balance should be maintained as outlined above (SaO_2 70–80%). Air or a means of delivering a low FiO_2 will usually be required during transfer to and from operating theater and ICU.

- Line sites should be aimed to be preserved as much as possible.
- A single lumen jugular SVC line should be placed for mixed venous saturation measurement.
- Useful physiological information is obtained when the shunt/PA conduit is unclamped toward the end of bypass. A fall in perfusion pressure of more than 25–30 mm Hg implies high Qp, and steps should be taken to increase PVR by immediately reducing FiO_2 and allowing CO_2 to rise during the wean from bypass.
- Echocardiogram should be performed in the theater if unstable.

POSTOPERATIVE MANAGEMENT OF NORWOOD STAGE 1

Physiologically, infants are similar after a Norwood I procedure. The arterial duct has been replaced by a systemic-pulmonary artery shunt but both pulmonary and systemic circulations continue to be fed from a common source and the balance of PVR and SVR continues to determine the pulmonary and systemic flow ratio.

BALANCING SHUNTS POSTOPERATIVELY

Excessive Pulmonary Blood Flow

- Saturation >80% and PaO_2 >45 mm Hg suggests Qp: Qs >1.
- Low systemic diastolic pressure:
  - Nurse in air.
  - Correct any metabolic alkalosis (acetazolamide or arginine hydrochloride):
    - Elective hypoventilation to increase CO_2 to reduce Qp.
    - Lower ventilator rate but maintain tidal volume.
    - Add dead space to ventilator/tube interface to increase CO_2 rebreathing.
  - Increase PEEP.
  - Adding CO_2 is potentially dangerous and no longer recommended.
  - If evidence of excessive pulmonary blood flow persists despite the above measures give urgent consideration to insertion of a smaller shunt/PA conduit band.

Low Pulmonary Blood Flow

- Saturation <70% suggests Qp: Qs <1.
- Confirm shunt patency on echo.
- Exclude pulmonary causes of desaturation.
- Detect and correct systemic venous desaturation/low cardiac OP.

- Maintain high SVR by using systemic vasoconstrictor (noradrenaline 0.05-0.4 mg/kg/min) to "push" blood through the shunt/lungs.
- Decrease PVR—raise FiO_2.
- Induce alkalosis.
- Abolish vasoconstricting influences.
- Emergency surgery revision may be required if flow is very poor.
- Provided that a (small) shunt is patent, lower oxygen saturations (60-70%) may be acceptable in the early period postoperatively but saturations below 60%, especially if associated with acidosis or evidence of impaired systemic oxygen delivery, are unacceptable.
- *The interpretation of Qp:* Qs ratio using only systemic saturation assumes that mixed venous blood returning to the heart is saturated at approximately 50% and is unaltered by "balancing" maneuvers. This is rarely the case. Obtain a better understanding of the distributions of shunt flows and the (in) adequacy of systemic blood flow from serial measurement of SVC (but not atrial) saturation. A number of worked examples illustrating commonly encountered conditions are given.

Shunt Calculation

$$\frac{Qp}{Qs} = \frac{S_aO_2 - S_{SVC}O_2}{S_{pv}O_2 - S_{pa}O_2}$$

S_aO_2 = Systemic arterial oxygen saturation

$S_{SVC}O_2$ = Superior vena caval saturation

$S_{pv}O_2 / S_{pa}O_2$ = Pulmonary vein/artery saturations

In parallel circuits $S_aO_2 = S_{pa}O_2$ and can be assumed to be 95-100%.

Appendices

Appendix 1

Drug, Dilution, Administration and Dose

DRUG DOSAGES IN PEDIATRIC CARDIAC INTENSIVE CARE UNIT (PCICU)

Formula for calculating the inotropes:

$$\text{ML} = \frac{\text{Weight (kg)} \times 3 \times \text{Desired micrograms}}{\text{Strength}}$$

$$\text{ML} = \frac{\text{Weight (kg)} \times \text{Desired micrograms} \times 60 \times \text{Dilution}}{\text{Strength} \times 1000}$$

INOTROPES

Name	Strength	Dilution	Dose
Injection Dopamine	200 mg/5 mL	<10 kg: 50 mg in 50 mL NS 10–20 kg: 100 mg in 50 mL NS 20–40 kg: 200 mg in 50 mL NS >40 kg: 400 mg in 50 mL NS	2.5–15 µg/kg/mt
Injection Dobutamine	250 mg/5 mL	<10 kg: 125 mg in 50 mL NS >10 kg: 250 mg in 50 mL NS	2.5–15 µg/kg/mt
Injection Adrenaline	1 mg/mL	<10 kg: 1.5 mg/50 mL NS >10 kg: 3 mg/50 mL NS	0.01–3 µg/kg/mt
Injection Noradrenaline	4 mg/2 mL	<10 mg: 2 mg/20 mL NS >10 kg: 4 mg/50 mL NS	0.01–0.3 µg/kg/mt
Injection Milrinone	10 mg/10 mL	<10 kg: 5 mg/50 mL NS >10 kg: 10 mg/50 mL NS	0.25–0.75 µg/kg/mt
Injection Phenylephrine HCl (Frenin)	1 mL/10 mg	10 mg dilute in 10 mL: 1 mL = 1 mg	0.1–0.5 µg/kg/mt

CHRONOTROPES

Name	Strength	Dilution	Dose
Injection Isuprel	2 mg/1 mL	<10 kg: 2 mg/50 mL NS >10 kg: 4 mg/50 mL NS	0.01–0.3 μg/kg/mt

VASODILATORS

Name	Strength	Dilution	Dose
Injection Glyceryl Trinitrate (NTG)	25 mg/5 mL	<10 kg: 12.5 mg/50 mL of NS 10–20 kg: 25 mg/50 mL of NS >20 kg: 50 mg/50 mL of NS	1–10 μg/kg/mt
Injection Sodium Nitroprusside (SNP)	50 mg vial	<10 kg: 12.5 mg/50 mL of NS 10–20 kg: 25 mg/50 mL of NS >20 kg: 50 mg/50 mL of NS	0.5–10 μg/kg/mt
Injection Phenoxybenzamine	100 mg/2 mL	1 mg/kg dilute in 24 mL NS	0.5–1 mg/kg/mt

NARCOTICS

Name	Strength	Dilution	Dose
Injection Fentanyl	100 µg/2 mL 500 µg/10 mL	<10 kg: 10 µg/1cc = 100 µg/10 mL NS 10–20 kg: 25 µg/cc = 250 µg/10 mL NS >20 kg: 50 µg/cc = 500 µg/10 mL NS	1–2 µg–1 kg (Bolus) 1–4 µg/kg/h (Infusion)
Injection Morphine	10 mg/mL	<10 kg: 0.5 mg/cc = 5 mg in 10 mL NS >10 kg: 1 mL/cc = 10 mg in 10 mL NS	0.1–0.2 mg/kg (Bolus) 10–40 µg/kg/h (Infusion)

MUSCLE RELAXANTS

Name	Strength	Dilution	Dose
Injection Norcuron	10 mg vial	<10 kg: 5 mg in 10 mL = 0.5 mg/cc >10 kg: 10 mg in 10 mL = 1 mg/cc	0.1 mg/kg
Injection Pavulon	4 mg/2 mL	<10 kg: 2 mg in 4 mL = 0.5 mg/cc 10 to 20 kg: 4 mg in 4 mL = 1 mg/cc >20 kg: 2 mg/cc	0.1 mg/kg

LOOP DIURETICS

Name	Strength	Dilution	Dose
Injection Lasix	20 mg/2 mL	<10 kg: 10 mg in 2 mL = 5 mg/cc >10 kg: 20 mg in 2 mL = 10 mg/cc	0.5 mg–1 mg/kg (Bolus)
Tablet Lasix	40 mg–1 tab		0.5–1 mg/kg/dose BD
Tablet Aldactone	25 mg–1 tab		0.5–1 mg/kg/dose BD
Syrup Furoped	Dilute in 10 mL 30 mL bottle	1 mL = 10 mg	0.5–1 mg/kg/dose BD

OSMOTIC DIURETICS

Name	Strength	Dose
Injection Mannitol	20% (20 g in 100 mL)	0.25–0.5 g/kg/dose
Tablet Acetazolamide	250 mg	5–10 mg/kg/dose 6–8 hourly
Oral Glycerol	10%	1–1.8 g/kg/dose

ANTICONVULSANTS

Name	Strength	Dilution	Dose
Injection Diazepam	10 mg/2 mL	10 mg/10 mL	0.1–0.4 mg/kg/dose
Injection Midazolam	10 mg/10 mL	<10 kg: 5 mg/10 mL = 0.5 mg/cc >10 kg: 5 mg/5 mL = 1 mg/cc	0.1–0.2 mg/kg/dose
Injection Phenytoin Sodium	10 mg/2 mL	100 mg/10 mL	15–20 mg/kg/30 min (Loading) 3–5 mg/kg 12 hourly
Injection Phenobarbitone	200 mg/1 mL	200 mg/10 mL	15–20 mg/kg 30 min (Loading) 3–5 mg/kg/12 hourly

ELECTROLYTES

Name			Correct deficiency/Dose
Injection Calcium Gluconate 10% (1 mL = 98 mg)			0.2 ml/kg IV: maximum 10 mL or 10–20 mg/kg Deficit correction: 2 mL/kg/day
Injection Pottassium Chloride			0.3 mEq/kg slow IV
Injection Glucose D25			2 ml/kg/dose
Injection Sodium Bicarbonate (7.5%)			$$\text{Half} = \frac{\text{Base excess (BE) deficit} \times \text{Wt}}{6}$$
1 AMP (25 mL) = 22.3 mEq			$$\text{Full correction} = \frac{\text{BE deficit} \times \text{Wt}}{3}$$

BRONCHODILATORS

Name	Strength	Dilution	Dose
Injection Terbutaline	500 µg/1 mL	500 µg/20 mL	3–6 µg/kg/hourly (Loading) 0.4–1 µg/kg/min (Infusion)
Injection Aminophylline	250 mg/10 mL	125 mg/25 mL	5 mg/kg/over 30 min (Loading) 1 mg/kg/hourly (Infusion)
Injection Deriphylline	170 mg/2 mL		2 mg/kg/dose (Slow)

COAGULANTS

Name	Strength	Dilution	Dose
Injection Protamine Sulfate	50 mg/5 mL	10 mg/10 mL	1 mg/kg/dose
Injection Vitamin K	10 mg/1 mL	10 mg/10 mL	0.3 mg/kg/dose

Drug, Dilution, Administration and Dose

ANTICOAGULANTS

Name	Strength	Dilution	Dose
Injection Heparin	25,000 IU/5 mL	Infusion: 2500/50	5–15 IU/kg/hourly
Tablet Warfarin Sodium	5 mg: 1 tablet	5/10 smaller babies	0.2 mg/kg/once a day
Injection Clexane	20 mg, 40 mg, 60 mg		0.5 mg/kg/12 hourly SC

STEROIDS

Name	Strength	Dilution	Dose
Injection Decadron	8 mg/2 mL	<10 kg: 4 mg/2 mL = 2 mg/cc >10 kg: 8 mg/2 mL = 4 mg/cc	0.1–0.2 mg/kg/dose
Injection Hydrocortisone	100 mg vial	<10 kg: 50 mg/10 mL = 5 mg/cc >10 kg: 100 mg/10 mL = 10 mg/cc	2–4 mg/kg/dose
Injection Solumetrol	10 mg vial		2–4 mg/kg/dose
Tablet Prednisolone	10 mg, 20 mg		1–2 mg/kg 8th hourly

ANTIARRHYTHMICS

Name	Strength	Dilution	Dose
Injection Magnesium Sulfate	2 mL–50% 1 mL = 500 mg	Undiluted	0.2 mL/kg/dose/over 30 min 30 mg–50 mg/kg/dose over 30 min
Injection Adenosine	6 mg/2 mL	Undiluted	0.1–0.3 mg/kg/dose
Injection Amiodarone	150 mg/3 mL	150/50 mL <10 kg 50 mg/10 mL = 5 mg/cc	5 mg/kg over 1 hour followed by 5 μg/kg/min increase up to 25 μg/kg/min 5–15 μg/kg/min infusion (Maintenance)

Name	Strength	Dilution	Dose
Tablet Amiodarone	200 mg		4 mg/kg/dose 8th hourly
Injection Lignocaine (2%)	21.3 mg/mL	21.3/10—bolus 5 mL/20—infusion	1 mg/kg/dose 15–50 μg/kg/min
Injection Digoxin	500 μg/2 mL	500 μg/10 mL	5 μg/kg/12th hourly
Injection Atropine	0.6 mg/mL	0.6 mg/6 mL = 0.1 mg/cc	0.02 mg/kg/dose

ANTIHYPERTENSIVES

Name	Strength	Dilution	Dose
Tablet Captopril	250 mg	25 mg/10 mL	Test dose: 0.1 mg/kg 0.5 mg/kg 8th hourly
Tablet Enalapril	2.5 mg, 5 mg		Test dose: 0.1 mg/kg, 0.5 mg/kg 12th hourly

ANTACIDS

Name	Strength	Dilution	Dose
Injection Pantaprozole	40 mg/1 vial		0.8 mg/kg/once a day
Injection Ranitidine	50 g/2 mL	50 mg/10 mL	1 mg/kg/8th hourly
Tablet Ranitidine	150 mg		2–4 mg/kg/12th hourly
Syrup Sucralfate	1 g/10 mL		0–2 years: 2½ mL 6th hourly 2–12 years: 5 mL 6th hourly >12 years: 10 mL 6th hourly

SEDATIVES

Name	Strength	Dose
Syrup Triclofos (Pedicloryl)	500 mg/5 mL	75 mg/kg/dose
Injection Ketamine	500 mg/10 mL	2–4 mg/kg/dose 4 µg/kg/min—infusion

ANTIEMETICS

Name	Strength	Dose
Injection Metoclopramide (Perinorm)	10 mg/2 mL	0.15–0.3 mg/kg/day
Injection Emeset	4 mg/2 mL	0.2 mg/kg/dose 6–12th hourly
Tablet Emeset	1 tablet: 4 mg	0.1 mg/kg/dose
Injection Phenergan	25 mg/mL	0.1 to 0.3 mg/kg/dose 0.5 mg/kg/dose IV (Sedation)
Syrup Domstal		0.2–0.4 mg/kg/dose TDS
Syrup Emeset	2 mg/5 mL	0.1–0.2 mg/kg/dose 6–12th hourly

REVERSAL DRUGS

Name	Strength	Dose
Injection Naloxone	400 µg/mL	0.1 mg/kg/stat 0.01 mg/kg/hour
Injection Neostigmine	0.5 mg/1 mL	0.05–0.07 mg/kg/dose
Injection Glycopyrrolate	500 µg/5 mL	5–10 µg/kg/dose
Injection Myopyrolate	0.5 mg/5 mL	0.01 mg/kg/dose

ANTIPYRETICS

Name	Strength	Dose
Injection Paracetamol	1000 mg/100 mL	7.5 mg/kg/dose
Tablet Paracetamol	500 mg	10–15 mg/kg/dose 6–8th hourly
Syrup Paracetamol	120 mg/5 mL	10–15 mg/kg/dose 6–8th hourly
Syrup P–125	125 mg/5 mL	10–15 mg/kg/dose 6–8th hourly
Syrup P–250	250 mg/5 mL	10–15 mg/kg/dose 6–8th hourly
Dolo Drops	100 mg/1 mL	10–15 mg/kg/dose 6–8th hourly
Anamol Suppository	80 mg, 170 mg	10–15 mg/kg/dose 6–8th hourly

ANALGESICS

Name	Strength	Dose
Injection Tramadol	100 mg/2 mL	2 mg/kg/dose
Justin Suppository	12.5 mg, 100 mg	2 mg/kg/dose
Tablet Combiflam	200 mg, 400 mg	
Syrup Ibugesic Plus (60 mL)	Ibuprofen: 100 mg/5 mL Paracetamol: 162.5 mg/mL	

PULMONARY HYPERTENSION

Name	Strength	Dose
Tablet Bosentan	62.5 mg	1-2 mg/kg/dose 12th hourly
	120 mg	2 mg/kg/dose 12th hourly
Tab Sildenafil	20 mg	0.3 mg/kg/dose 6th hourly Max: 2–3 mg/kg/dose
Injection Phenoxybenzamine	1 mg/kg in 24 mL NS	0.5–1 µg/kg/mt

HEMATINICS

Name	Strength	Dose
Syrup Mumfer	50 mg/5 mL	3–5 mg/kg/day
Capsule Fesovit	33 mg/5 mL	6 mg/kg/12 hourly
Syrup Tonoferon	250 mg/5 mL	6 mg/kg/12 hourly

MISCELLANEOUS

Name	Strength	Dilution	Dose
GIK			0.5 mL/kg/hourly
GI Bolus		25D 9.9 mL: 0.1 mL	0.1 IU/kg/IV
Syrup Osteocalcium	82 mg/5 mL		>1 year: 1 tsp 12th hourly
Injection Prostaglandin E1	500 µg/mL		0.01–0.1 µg/kg/min
Injection Immunoglobulin	0.5 g, 1 g	Undiluted	400 mg/kg/dose
Injection Avil (Pheniramine)	22.7 mg/mL		0.2 to 0.4 mg/kg/day

Contd...

Contd...

Name	Strength	Dilution	Dose
Syrup S–Mucolite	15 mg/5 mL (60 mL)		Child <2 years: 7.5 mg BID 2–5 years: 7.5 mg BID/TID 6–12 years: 15 mg BID/TID
Syrup Allegra (Fexofenadine)	30 mg/5 mL (60 mL)		<12 years: 30 mg TDS >12 years: 60 mg TDS

LAXATIVES

Name	Strength	Dose
Tablet Dulcolax	5 mg	<5 years 5–10 mg HS >5 years 10–20 mg HS
Suppository	5 mg, 10 mg	<12 months: 2.5 mg >12 months: 5 mg Adult: 10 mg
Syrup Lactulose	10 g/15 mL	0.5 mL/kg/dose
Proctoclysis (Enema)		Children: 10 mL to 20 mL Adult: 100 mL

NEBULIZING AGENTS

Name	Dose
Asthalin	0.15 mg/kg/dose
Budecort	<12 years: 50–200 µg 6–12th hourly >12 years: 100–600 µg 6–12th hourly
Ipravent	250 µg in 2–4 mL NS 6–8th hourly
Mucomix (N-acetylcysteine)	0.1 mL/kg/dose: 6–12th hourly 10%–0.1 mL; 20%–0.05 mL
Adrenaline: 1:1000	0.05 mL/kg/dose in 4 mL 4–6th hourly
Levosalbutamol	0.63 mg ½ respule 6–8th hourly
Inhalex: 7.5 mg 15 mg	<5 years ½ respule 12th hourly >5 years 1 respule 12th hourly

Drug, Dilution, Administration and Dose

ANTIBIOTICS AMINOGLYCOSIDES

Name	Strength	Dilution	Dose
Injection Amikacin	250 mg–500 mg/2 mL	250/10, 500/10	7.5 mg/kg/dose 12th hourly
Injection Garamicin	80 mg/2 mL	80 mg/10 mL	2.5 mg/kg/dose 12th hourly
Injection Netilmicin	100 mg, 200 mg, 300 mg	100 mg/10 mL 200 mg/10 mL 300 mg/10 mL	8 mg/kg/dose 1st 24 hours, 2–6 mg/kg/24 hours

CEPHALOSPORINES

Name	Strength	Dose
Injection Cefuroxime	250 mg, 750 mg	30 mg/kg/dose 8th hourly
Injection Cefazolin	1 g vial	30 mg/kg/dose 8th hourly
Injection Cefotamine	1 g vial	50 mg/kg/dose 8th hourly
Injection Ceftriaxone	1 g vial	50 mg/kg/dose 8th hourly
Injection Ceftazidime	1 g vial	50 mg/kg/dose 8th hourly
Injection Cefipime	1 g vial	50 mg/kg/dose 8th hourly
Injection Cepirome	1 g vial	50 mg/kg/dose 12th hourly
Injection Ceftizoxime	1 g vial	50 mg/kg/dose 6–8th hourly
Injection Magnex	1 g vial	50 mg/kg/dose 8th hourly

FLUOROQUINOLONES

Name	Strength	Dose
Injection Ciprofloxacin	200 mg/100 mL	8 mg/kg/dose 12th hourly
Injection Ofloxacin	200 mg/100 mL	8 mg/kg/dose 12th hourly

PENICILLIN GROUP

Name	Strength	Dilution	Dose
Injection Augmentin	300 mg, 1.2 g	300 mg/10 mL	30 mg/kg/dose 8th hourly
Injection Ampicillin	500 mg vial	500 mg/10 mL	50 mg/kg/dose 6–8th hourly

ANTIFUNGAL

Name	Strength	Dilution	Dose
Injection Fluconazole	200 mg/100 mL	Undiluted	6 mg/kg/day (Single dose)
Injection Itraconazole	200 mg, 400 mg		4 mg/kg/dose 12th hourly

MISCELLANEOUS

Name	Strength	Dilution	Dose
Injection Ticloplanin	200 mg, 400 mg	Dose in 10 mL (30 min)	10 mg/kg/dose 12th hourly × 3 doses OD
Injection Imipenem	500 mg	500 mg/10 mL	25 mg/kg/dose 8th hourly
Injection Meropenem	500 mg	500 mg/10 mL	20 mg/kg/dose 8th hourly (Max—40 mg/kg)
Injection Zosyn	4.2 g		50 mg/kg/dose 6th hourly (Max—75 mg/kg)
Injection Linezolid	400 mg	400 mg/10 mL	10 mg/kg/dose 8th hourly (Max—75 mg/kg)
Injection Metrogyl	500 mg/100 mL	Undiluted	7.5 mg/kg/dose 8th hourly
Injection Vancomycin	500 mg	500 mg/10 mL	10–15 mg/kg/dose 6–8th hourly

Appendix 2

Flowcharts

Suryanarayanpillai Hari Prakash

Flowchart A2.1: Mild-to-moderate hypotension.

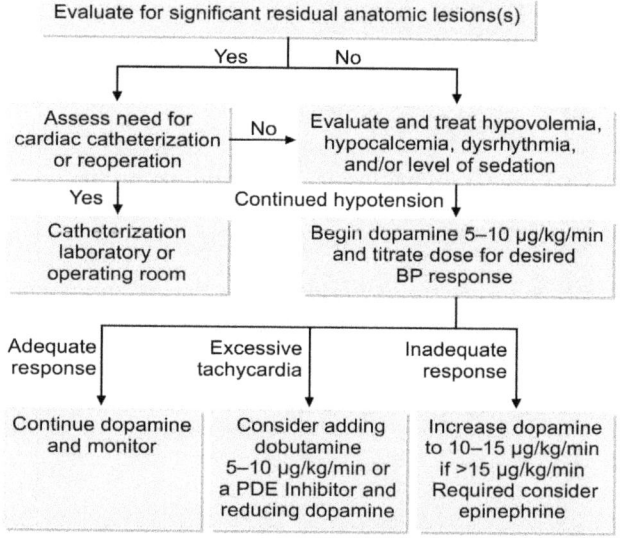

Flowchart A2.2: Normal or mildly decreased BP with low CO and elevated SVR.

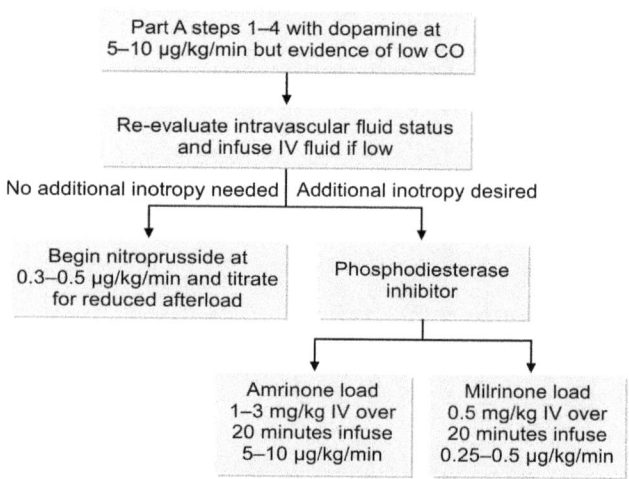

Flowchart A2.3: Severe hypotension.

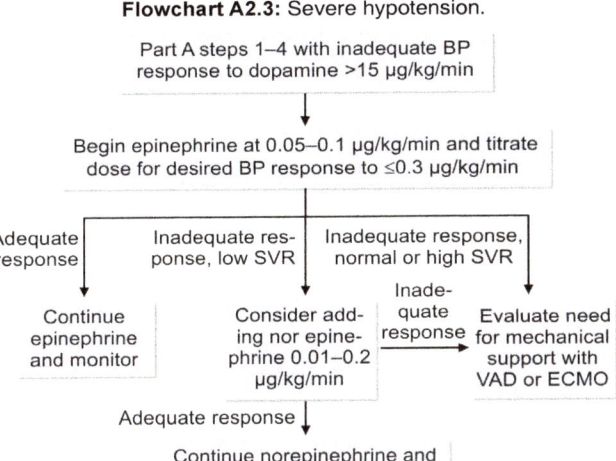

Flowchart A2.4: Management of postextubation stridor.

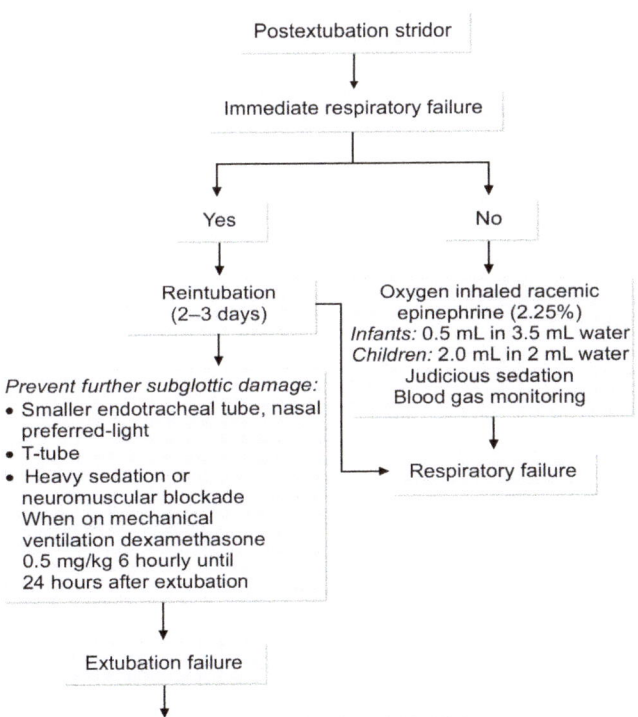

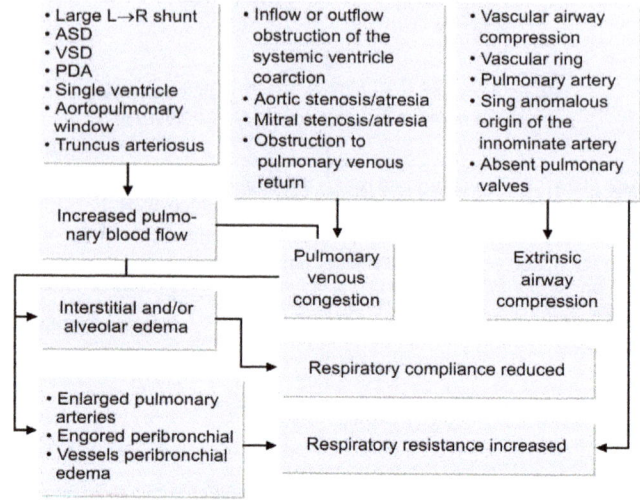

Flowchart A2.5: Alteration of respiratory mechanics by cardiac anomalies.

Flowchart A2.6: Diagnosis and management of chylothorax.

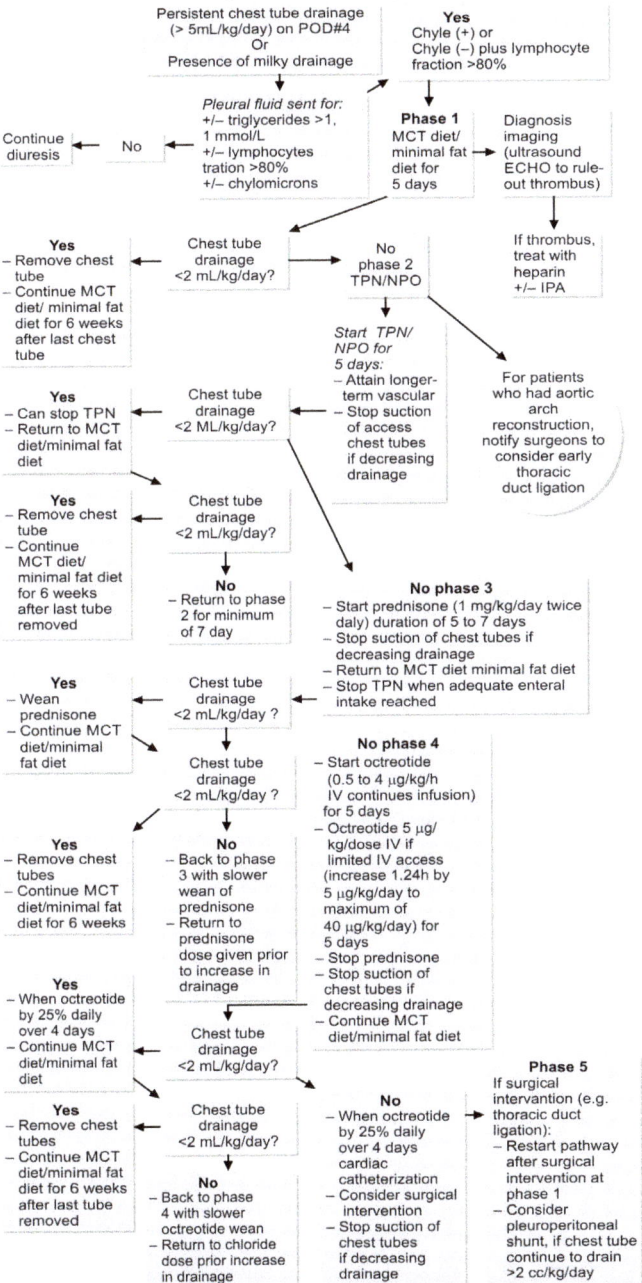

(ECHO: echocandiogram; IV: intravenous; MCT: medium chain triglycerides formula or nutritional supplement; NPO: nothing by mouth; POD: postoperative day; Q8h: 8th hourly; q24h: daily; tPA: tissue plasminogen activator; TPN: total parenteral nutrition)

Appendix 3

Guidelines for Endotracheal Suction

Prabhu Mayakesavan

GUIDELINES FOR ENDOTRACHEAL SUCTION PICU (ROYAL LIVERPOOL CHILDREN'S NHS TRUST)

Action	Rationale	Evidence
Endotracheal suction should only be performed when there are indications that increased pulmonary secretions are adversely affecting the ventilation of patients with artificial airways	Endotracheal suction is a potentially hazardous procedure that can adversely affect the ventilation of the patient with an artificial airway The known hazards of endotracheal suction are: • Arrhythmias/cardiac arrest • Hypoxia • Raised intracranial pressure • Hypo/hypertension • Trauma/pulmonary hemorrhage • Laryngospasm • Infection • Pain and discomfort • Pneumothorax • Retrolental fibroplasia	
Endotracheal suction should only be carried out by appropriately trained staff in an area equipped to deal with the emergency management of the airway	Staff should be constantly aware of the hazards of endotracheal suction, and should be skilled in the assessment of respiratory function and the management of airway/respiratory problems, to maintain the safety of patients with artificial airways	

Contd...

Contd...

Action	Rationale	Evidence
Indications of endotracheal suction	Endotracheal suction is a potentially hazardous procedure and should therefore only be performed when there is clear clinical indication for the presence of excessive pulmonary secretions affecting the patency of the artificial airway or the effective ventilation of the patient	
	Respiratory distress	
Changes in heart rate:	Hypoxia	
• Tachycardia		
• Bradycardia		
Decreased SaO_2	Hypoxia	Walsh CM, Bada HS, 1987
Increases in $ETCO_2$	CO_2 retention	
Deterioration in blood gas estimations	Hypoxia or hypercarbia from retained secretions	Fox WW Schwartz JG, 1978
Increases in $PaCO_2$	Postsuction hypoxia—derecruitment of alveoli	
Decreases in $PaCO_2$	Pulmonary edema	
Increased work of breathing	Respiratory distress	
Increased respiratory rate	Obstructed airway/secretions/hypoxia or hypercarbia	
Forced inspiration/expiration		

Appendix 4
Responsibilities of the Bedside Nurse when Chest Closing or Opening

K Mahalaxmi, R Kokila

BEFORE THE PROCEDURE

Management of the Patient

- Prepare the child and parents of the impending procedure.
- Ensure cross-matched blood is in the theater fridge.
- Ensure 10–20 mL sodium chloride flush, 10% calcium gluconate, fentanyl (or intensivists preference), midazolam and vecuronium syringes plus emergency drugs are near the intensivist.
- Connect Lectrocath with three-way tap (distal to the patient) to a lumen on the central line.
- Connect a 50 mL syringe of plasma to one end of the three-way tap.
- Connect, or ask doctor, pacing wires to appropriate pacing box.
- Place incontinence sheet under patient.
- Place diathermy pad under patient with theater staff.
- Ensure patient has had a bolus of sedation, analgesia, and vecuronium for the procedure.
- Place roll under neck.

Management of the Environment

- Clear cubicle of locker, green trolley, tables, chairs.
- If the patient is in a cot, obtain car jacks, and with the assistance of extra staff, place the cot on the jacks.
- Place defibrillator with appropriate internal connections and paddles plugged in cubicle.
- Place screens around the bedside.
- Arrange for light source for the surgeon.

DURING THE PROCEDURE

The role of the nurse is to act as "runner" for the theater staff.

AFTER THE PROCEDURE

The nurse must assess the patient at quarter-to-half hour intervals for signs of low cardiac output—cooling peripheries, reduction in urine output, tachycardia, low blood pressure and report promptly.

Management of the Environment

Return the bed space to a safe working environment.

Index

Page numbers followed by *f* refer to figure, *fc* refer to flowchart, and *t* refer to table

A

Acetazolamide 150
Acid-base management 86
Acidosis 16, 20, 21, 33, 66, 88, 94
    metabolic 20, 44
Activated partial thromboplastin time 7, 104, 108
Adenosine 57, 62, 154
Administer local antibiotic therapy 108
Adrenaline 132, 139, 147, 158
    nebulisation 79
Aerogenes 117
Airway 2, 4, 142
    humidification of 113
Albumin 7
    serum 77
Aldactone 150
Alpha-adrenergic agonists, administration of 88
Ambu bag 3
Amikacin 159
Amiloride 40
Aminoglycosides
    administration of 94
    antipseudomonal 119
    resist, high-level 117
Aminophylline 152
Amiodarone 57, 60, 62, 154
    infusion 59
Amoxicillin 118
    clavulanate 119
Ampicillin 117, 118, 160
    sulbactam 119
Amrinone 98, 99
Analgesia 91
Analgesics 30, 93, 157
Anesthesia 143
    local 72*f*
    management 124
Antacids 155
Antiacetylcholine esterase drugs 94
Antiarrhythmics 154
    administration of 94
Antibiotics 115
    aminoglycosides 159
    systemic 85
Anticoagulation, postoperative 103
Anticonvulsant 151
    therapy 87
Antiemetics 156
Antihypertensives 155
Anti-inflammatory drugs 121

Antimicrobial 114
    agent 117
Antipyretics 156
Aorta
    coarctation of 135, 135*f*
    overriding of 133
Aortic stenosis 136, 136*f*
Aortoplasty, subclavian 135
Appropriate suction catheter, formula for selection of 113
Arrhythmia 54, 88, 97, 99, 101, 102, 112, 114
    acute hemodynamically significant 62*t*
    cardiac 42, 54
    causes of 54
    types of 54
    ventricular 54, 97
Arterial blood gas 20
    analysis 29
Arterial ducts, artificial 122
Arterial pressure monitoring 8
Arterial pulse pressure 17
Arterial switch procedure 10, 138
Arterial vasodilatation 99
Arterial waveform 9*f*, 18
Artery
    forceps 72*f*
        straight 105
    pressure
        high pulmonary 126
        mean pulmonary 12
Ascites 18, 26
Aspiration 81
    gastric 106
Aspirin 103, 137
Asthalin 158
Atelectasis 81, 110
Atenolol 57
Atracurium 95
Atrial contraction, loss of 20
Atrial fibrillation 58, 103
Atrial filling pressures 18
Atrial fixed pacing 67
Atrial flutter 57
Atrial premature beat 56
Atrial rate 57
Atrial rhythm, low 54
Atrial septal defect 56, 103, 128, 129*f*
Atrioventricular canal defect 130, 131*f*
Atrioventricular nodal reentry tachycardia 54

Atrium 54
Atropine 62, 154
Augmentin 160
Avil 157
A-wave 11
Azithromycin 117, 118
Aztreonam 118

B

Bacteremia, primary 115
Bacteroides fragilis species 117
Balancing shunts
    postoperatively 144
    preoperatively 143
Balloon
    atrial septostomy 54
    tipped pulmonary flotation catheter 11
Benzodiazepines 92
Beta-blocker 57-59, 133
Betadine 106
Bilirubin, serum 7
Bipyridines 98
B-lactamase 117, 118
Bladder care 105
Blalock-Taussig shunt 80, 122, 122*f*
    modified 36
Bleeding 47, 49
    gastrointestinal 85
Blood
    count, full 115
    culture 115
    film 115
    flow
        excessive pulmonary 143, 144
        low pulmonary 143, 144
        pulmonary 23
        systemic 23
    gas targets, initial 142
    glucose 7, 37
    losses 38
    pressure 4, 22
        arterial 3, 9
        lower arterial 33
        mean arterial 12
        normal 22*t*
        systemic 37
        systolic 22
    products 38, 46, 47
    replacement 38
    sugar 37, 77
    transfusion, excessive 44
    urea 7
    urea nitrogen 19, 26, 37
Bordetella pertussis 117
Bosentan 157
Bowel care 105
Bradycardia 18, 33
Breath sounds, bilateral 29
Bretylium 60
Bronchoconstriction 42, 101
Bronchodilator 94, 152
Bronchoscopy 91
Bronchospasm 81, 83
Budecort nebulizer 83
Bundle of His 54, 58, 63
Burns 11, 40, 41

C

Calcium 44, 77
    chloride 44
    gluconate 39, 77, 151
    levels, low 42
    low ionized 20
    resonium 38
    sensitizer 101
Campylobacter 117
Canon waves 11
Capillary hydrostatic pressure 81
Capillary leak 18
    syndrome 52
Capnograph
    abnormal 14*f*
    normal 14*f*
Capnography 13
Captopril 155
Carbohydrates 77
Cardiac anomalies 164*fc*
Cardiac arrest 1
Cardiac catheterization 23
Cardiac decompression 20
Cardiac failure
    chronic congestive 99
    congestive 85
Cardiac index 19, 87
Cardiac intensive care unit 62*t*
Cardiac pacemakers 2
Cardiac surgery 86
Cardiac tamponade 20, 21, 45, 51
Cardiomyopathy 11, 58
    dilated 97
Cardiopulmonary bypass 1, 23, 35, 48, 99, 114, 133
Cardiovascular function 16
Cardiovascular management 16
Cardioversion 91
Carotid artery 11
Catecholamine
    excessive 54
    levels 93
Cavity, pleural 70
Cefadroxil 116

Cefazolin 116, 159
Cefepime 116, 159
Cefmetazole 116
Cefotamine 159
Cefotaxime 118
Cefotetan 116
Ceftazidime 119, 159
Ceftizoxime 159
Ceftriaxone 118, 159
Cefuroxime 116, 159
Central nervous system 2
    issues, postoperative 86
Central O_2 delivery 2
Central venous
    catheter 115
    oxygen saturation 19
    pressure 10, 10f, 12, 37, 100
Cephalosporines 159
    first-generation 116
    fourth-generation 116
    parental 119
    second-generation 116
    third-generation 116
Cephapirin 116
Cephradine 116
Cepirome 159
Cerebral
    edema 86
    embolization 86
    hypoperfusion 86
    perfusion 86
Chest
    drain 70, 91
        tubes 6
    physiotherapy 83
    radiography 121
    tube 70
        insertion of 72f, 80
    wall expansion 29
    X-ray 21, 123
Chlamydia
    pneumoniae 117
    trachomatis 117
Chloramphenicol 118
Chloride 77
Chloroxylenol 105
Cholestasis 77
Choreiform movements 86
Chronic obstructive airways
    disease 11
Chronotropes 148
Chylothorax 81
    diagnosis of 165fc
    management of 165fc
    medical management of 82
    surgical management of 82
Cilastatin 119

Ciprofloxacin 118, 119, 160
Cisapride 76
Citrate toxicity 46
Citrobacter diversus 117
Clarithromycin 118
Clexane 153
Clindamycin 117, 119
Cloacae 117
Clostridium
    difficile 117
    tetani 117
Cold blood 46
Coma 40, 41
Combiflam 157
Conduction disorders 64
Congestion, hepatic 45
Conscious sedation 92
Coronary artery, anomalous left
    7, 10, 139, 140f
Corticosteroids 121
Coumarin anticoagulation,
    emergency reversal
    of 49
Cramps, abdominal 101
C-reactive protein 114
Creatinine 37
Cryoprecipitate 46, 49
C-wave 11
Cyanide toxicity 99

D

Decadron 153
Decompression 80
Deep sedation 34
Delirium 41
Delta wave 59
Deriphylline 152
Desmopressin 47
Dexamethasone 32, 79
Dexmedetomidine 92
Dextran 37
Dextrose 101
Diabetes insipidus 40
Diarrhea 40-42
Diazepam 86, 87, 92, 151
DiGeorge syndrome 44
Digoxin 57, 61, 154
Dilantin 60
Dipyridamole 103
Distention, abdominal 31
Dithromycin 118
Diuretic therapy 40, 42
Dizziness 63
Dobutamine 24, 26, 97, 147
Dolo drops 156
Domperidone 76
Domstal 156

Dopamine 24, 94, 147
  high dose of 88
  low dose of 26
Down's syndrome 131
Doxycycline 117, 118
Dressler's syndrome 120
Drowsiness 41
Drug 147
Dulcolax 158
Dysarhythmias 8

E

Ebstein's anomaly 58, 59
Ebstein's malformation 56
Echocardiography 19, 21
  transesophageal 91
Ectopic tachycardia, junctional 22, 54, 58, 62
Edema
  generalized 26
  peripheral 26
  pulmonary 81
Edrophonium 94
Eisenmenger syndrome 129
Ejection fraction 19
Electrocardiogram 3, 8, 8*f*
  normal 55*f*
Electrolyte 77*t*, 151
  abnormalities 77
  disturbances 20
  imbalances 66
Emboli, systemic 103
Embolism 86
Emeset 156
Enalapril 155
Endocarditis 117
Endotracheal suction 33, 110, 112, 166
  hazards of 112
  preparing for 112
Endotracheal tube 2, 27, 107
  aspiration 115
  complications 79
  size 113
  selection of 28
End-tidal carbon dioxide 13, 19
  monitoring 13
Enema 158
Enoxacin 119
Enteral feeds 75
Enteral nutrition 75
Enterococcus faecalis 117
Enterocolitis, necrotizing 85
Epiglottitis 118
Epinephrine 25, 32, 62, 96
Epoprostenol 100
Erythrocyte sedimentation rate 114

Erythromycin 117-119
Escherichia coli 117
Esmolol 62
Exercise intolerance 63
Extracellular fluid volume 44
Extubation 31
  failure 80
Eye
  care of 108
  drops 108
  ointment 108

F

Facial pallor 101
Failure to thrive 130
Fatal tachycardia 91
Fatigue, diaphragmatic 31
Feeding 75
Fentanyl 34, 93, 149
Fever 114
Fexofenadine 158
Fick principle 11
Fistula, bronchopleural 81
Fits 42
Flucloxacillin prophylaxis 115
Fluconazole 160
Fluid 37
  and electrolyte management 35
  balance 90
  intravenous 35
  restriction 41
  types of 37
Fluoroquinolones 119, 160
Foley's catheters 2, 105
Fontan procedure 36, 58, 103, 127
  extracardiac 103, 127
Fresh frozen plasma 24, 37, 46, 48, 139
Furosemide 37, 88
Fungal organisms 85
Furoped 150
Furosemide, administration of 94

G

Garamycin 159
Gastrointestinal tract 135
Gentamicin 117, 118
Glenn flow 125
Glenn pressure 126
Glenn procedure 80
  bi-directional 103
Glenn shunt, bi-directional 124, 126
Glucose D25 151
  infusion rates 77
  serum 87

Glycerine suppository 1-5, 84
Glyceryl trinitrate 148
Glycopyrrolate 156
Great artery, transposition of 137, 138*f*

H

Haemophilus influenzae 115, 118
Headache 100
Heart
 block 16
  complete 21, 134
  second-degree 61
  third-degree 19, 63
 defect, congenital 122
 disease
  acyanotic 129, 130
  congenital 59, 61
  cyanotic congenital 132
  valvular 11
 failure 41, 101
 lesions, congenital 56
 rate 21, 65
  abnormalities of 18
  average 21, 21*t*
 sounds, fourth 19
 surgery
  closed 36
  open 36, 45
 valves, prosthetic 22
Hematinics 157
Hematocrit 35, 37, 47
Hemofiltration 90
Hemorrhage 86, 138
 pulmonary 112
Heparin 123, 153
 reversal of 47
Hepatic failure 49
Histamine-2-receptor antagonist 76
Hospital-acquired lower respiratory tract infection 115
Human albumin 50, 50*t*
 solutions 50
Hydration, adequate 113, 123
Hydrocortisone 153
Hypercapnia 94
Hypercarbia 21, 80
Hyperglycemia 41, 77, 89
Hyperkalemia 21, 38
Hyperlipidemia 41
Hypernatremia 40, 41*fc*
Hyperproteinemia 41
Hyperpyrexia, malignant 114
Hypertension 112
 pulmonary arterial 93, 97
 severe systemic 99
 venous 81
Hyperthermia 20, 54, 106, 107
 malignant 15
Hyperthyroidism 61
Hypertriglyceridemia 77
Hypertrophy 16, 26
 right ventricular 133
Hypocalcemia 21, 42, 44, 47
 causes of 44
 severe 44
Hypoglycemia 77, 88
Hypokalemia 21, 39, 42, 77, 84, 97, 101
Hyponatremia 41, 43*fc*
 causes of 42*fc*
Hypophosphatemia 77
Hypoplastic left heart syndrome 140
Hypotension 58, 60, 80, 97, 100, 101, 112
 development of 16
 mild-to-moderate 162*fc*
 severe 163*fc*
 systemic arterial 24
Hypothermia 45, 54, 88, 94
Hypoventilation 20
Hypovolemia 18, 23, 24
Hypoxemia 80, 81*t*, 97
Hypoxia 21, 54, 66, 81, 88, 112

I

Ibugesic plus 157
Icterus 84
Imipenem 119, 161
Immunoglobulin 157
Infarction, gastric 101
Infection 112
 issues 114
 prevention of 77
Inflammatory febrile condition 120
Infusion pumps 2
Inhalex 158
Inodilator 101
Inotropes 96, 102*t*
Intercostal catheters, insertion of 71
Intermittent mandatory ventilation mode 31
Intra-aortic balloon pump 139
Intracranial pressure, raised 112
Intubation 133
 several days of 31
Invasive monitoring devices 8
Ipratropium 83
Ipravent 158

Ischemia 8, 11
  myocardial 54, 97, 101, 138
  postoperative 18
  reperfusion injury 35
Isoproterenol 25, 62, 98
Isuprel 148
Itraconazole 160

J

Jaundice 84
Jugular vein
  external 10
  internal 10

K

Ketamine 94, 156
Ketoacidosis, diabetic 42
Kidney 2
Klebsiella pneumoniae 118

L

Lactate, serum 19
Lactulose 158
Lansoprazole 76
Laryngomalacia 79
Laryngoscope 2
Laryngospasm 112
Lasix 150
Leads 64
Left atrial
  catheters 9
  line 9
  pressure 12, 37
Left atrium 17
Left bundle branch block 55
Left ventricular
  stroke work index 12
  volume 9, 12
Leptospira interrogans 118
Lethargy 40, 41
Leukocytosis 121
Levosalbutamol 158
Levosimendan 101
Lidocaine 60, 62
Lignocaine 73, 154
Linezolid 118, 161
Listeria monocytogenes 118
Lithium dilution 19
Liver 2
  failure 41
  function tests 7, 77
Lomefloxacin 119
Loop diuretics 150
Lorazepam 87, 92
Low cardiac output 20, 114
  signs of 24
  state 18t
    assessment of 17
  syndrome 101
Lymphangiography 82

M

Magnesium 77
  deficiency 42
  depletion, causes of 42
  levels, low 42
  sulfate 62, 154
Magnex 159
Mannitol 150
Massive air leak 80
Mechanical ventilation 30, 80
Mediastinal bleeding 45
  management of 45
Mediastinitis 121
Mediastinum 70
Medium chain triglycerides
    formula 165
Meningitis 117, 118
Meningococcus 118
Mental status 18
Menthol 105
Meropenem 119, 161
Metaraminol 133
Metoclopramide 76, 156
Metrogyl 161
Metronidazole 117
Microvascular bleeding, treatment
    of 49
Midazolam 30, 87, 92, 151
Milliamperes 66
Milrinone 26, 33, 99, 132, 147
Minimal enteral nutrition 77
Mitral valve disease 11
Morphine 30, 93, 133, 149
Moxalactam 116
Mucomix 158
Multiorgan failure 85
Mumfer 157
Muscle relaxants 30, 94, 149
  nondepolarizing 94
Mycoplasma 118
Myocardial dysfunction 18
Myocardial protection,
    suboptimal 16
Myocarditis 97
Myopyrolate 156

N

N-acetylcysteine 158
Naloxone 156
Narcotics 149
Nasal endotracheal tube, routine
    care of 107

Nasogastric feeding 75, 105
Nasogastric tube 2, 84, 106
Nausea 41, 101
Near-infrared spectroscopy regional oxygen saturation 19
Neisseria meningitidis 118
Neonatal cardiac transplantation 140
Neostigmine 94, 156
Nephritic syndrome 41
Netilmicin 159
Nitric oxide 34
Nitroglycerine 100
Nitroprusside 99
Nodal bradycardia 21
Noninvasive continuous positive airway pressure 79
Noradrenaline 147
  infusion 133
Norcuron 149
Norepinephrine 97
Normothermia 32
Norwood stage, postoperative management of 144
Nutrition 75

O

Obstructive lesions 18
Ofloxacin 117-119, 160
Oliguria 16, 20
Omeprazole 76
Opioids 30, 93
Oral antacids 84
Oral endotracheal tube, routine care of 107
Oral feeds 105
Oral glycerol 150
Orotracheal route 28
Osmotic diuretics 40, 150
Osteocalcium 157
Otitis media 115
Oxygen 20*fc*, 133
  humidified 32
  saturation, mixed venous 11, 19
  supplemental 27
Oxygenation 12
  criteria 30

P

P wave axis 56
Pacemaker 64
  display 65*f*
  epicardial 64
  temporary 64
  transcutaneous external 64
  transvenous endocardial 64
Packed cell volume 51, 139
Packed red blood cells 47
Pain management 91
Pancuronium 30, 95
Pantaprozole 84, 155
Paracetamol 114, 156
Paralysis, diaphragmatic 80
Parenteral nutrition 76
Paresis 31, 80
Paresthesiae 42
Partial thromboplastin time 45
Patent ductus arteriosis 103
Pavulon 149
Pediatric cardiac
  intensive care unit 1, 147
  management, special features of 16
Pedicloryl 156
Pefloxacin 118, 119
Penicillin
  antipseudomonal 119
  G 117-119
  group 160
  V 119
Penicillinase-resistant synthetic penicillins 119
Pericardial tamponade 22
Pericardiocentesis 91
Pericardium 70
Perinorm 156
Peritoneal dialysis 2, 88, 89
  cycles 90
Peritonitis 41
Phenergan 156
Pheniramine 157
Phenobarbitone 87, 151
Phenoxybenzamine 33, 100, 148, 157
Phenylephrine 147
Phenytoin sodium 151
Phosphodiesterase inhibitors 98
Phosphorus 77
Phrenic nerve lesions 80
Physiotherapy 110, 112
Piperacillin 119
Platelet 48
  count 45
  transfusion 46, 48
Pleural fluid
  analysis 82
  aspiration 73
Pleurectomy 81
  surgical 83
Pleurodesis 81, 83
Pleuroperitoneal shunt 82

Pneumonia 118
Pneumothorax 80, 81
Polyuria 40
Positive end-expiratory pressure 4, 29, 31, 53
Postextubation
    stridor, management of 163*fc*
    subglottic edema 79
Postoperative pain, management of 91
Postpericardiotomy syndrome 120
Postural drainage 111, 111*f*
Potassium 37, 47, 77
    chloride 37, 151
    correction of 84
    serum 39*f*
Prednisolone 153
Pressure
    control ventilator 28, 29
    intracranial 100
    suction, low 70
Procainamide 60, 62
Proctoclysis 158
Prokinetic agents 76
Propranolol 133
Prostacyclin 100
Prostaglandin E1 157
    low dose 142
Prosthetic valve 137
    replacement 103
Protamine sulfate 47, 152
Protein 7, 76
    requirements, age-related 76*t*
Proteus mirabilis 118
Prothrombin time 7, 45, 108
Proton pump inhibitor 76
Pseudomonas aeruginosa 118
Pulmonary artery 7, 10, 19, 125, 139, 140*f*
    banding 126, 126*f*
    catheters 11
    occlusion pressure 11
    pressure 11, 33, 37, 100
Pulmonary capillary wedge pressure 100
Pulmonary hypertension 11, 18, 25, 33, 42, 129, 157
    crisis 33
    management 33
Pulmonary vascular resistance 12, 91, 97, 141
Pulse
    contour analysis 19
    generator 64
    oximeter oxygen saturations 3
    oximetry 12
Pulsus paradoxus 51
Pyridazone dinitrile derivative 101
Pyridostigmine 94

Q

QRS complex narrow 56

R

Radiofrequency ablation 57, 58
Ranitidine 76, 84, 155
Rapid atrial depolarization 57
Red cell, transfusion of 45
Regional oxygen saturation 19
Reintubation 79
Renal failure 44, 88
Renal function 19
Renal system 88
Renal tubular dysfunction 41
Respiratory
    assessment 27
    distress syndrome, acute 11, 81
    infection 33
    management 27
    mechanics, alteration of 164*fc*
    monitoring 12
    rate 12, 29
        spontaneous 27
    status 18
    tract infection, lower 115
Resuscitation, alveolar rupture 80
Rheumatic disease, severe 58
Rhythm, abnormalities of 18
Rifampin 117-119
Right atrial pressure 10, 37
    lowers 53
Right atrium 17
    pressure 33
Right bundle branch block 54, 134
Right ventricle 25
Right ventricular
    assist device 26
    dysfunction 10, 12
    failure 45
    outflow tract 133
Right ventriculotomy incisions 26
Rocuronium 95
Ross procedure 137
Rule of ten 89

S

Salbutamol bolus 38
Saline bullets 109
Salmonella typhi 118
Sedation 91, 133
    adequate 91
Sedatives 30, 92, 156

Seizure 40, 41, 86, 87
   etiology 86
Seldinger technique 10
Sense indicator 66
Sepsis 11, 33, 85, 114
   less common 114
   line-related 115
Seroma 124
Serratia marcescens 118
Serum electrolytes 37, 82, 87
   measurements 37
Serum glutamic oxaloacetic transaminase 7
Setting up synchronized intermittent mandatory ventilation 29, 30
Shock
   cardiogenic 99
   hyperdynamic septic 97
   septic 99
Sildenafil 157
Sinus 21
   arrhythmia 56
   bradycardia 54, 55
   rhythm 26
      normal 54
   tachycardia 54
Sinusitis 115
Skin care 108
Sodabicarb 88
Sodium 47, 77
   bicarbonate 151
   intake, high 40
   nitroprusside 148
   polystyrene sulfonate 38
Solumetrol 153
Staphylococcus
   aureus 114, 118
   epidermidis 114
Stenosis 33
   infundibular 133
   pulmonary 11
   residual pulmonary 26
   severe aortic 137
   subglottic 79
Sterile disposable syringes 73
Steroid 153
   role of 53
   therapy, systemic 83
Stethoscope 2
Stoma care 109
Streptococcus
   milleri 119
   pneumoniae 119
   pyogenes 119
Stress
   chronic 99
   response 114
   ulcers 84, 85

Stridor 79
Stroke volume index 12
Sucralfate 84, 85, 155
Suction catheter 2
   size of 113
Sulfamethoxazole 119
Superior vena cava 19, 122
Supracardiac total anomalous pulmonary venous connection 132*f*
Surgery 143
   timing of 143
Swan-Ganz catheter 17
Synchrony, atrioventricular 54
Syncope 63
Synchronized intermittent mandatory ventilation 29
Syringe pumps 2

T

Tachyarrhythmia 98
   supraventricular 22
Tachycardia 18, 51, 56, 58, 80, 98, 129
   atrial 54
   supraventricular 56, 62
Tachypnea 129
Tazobactam 119
Teicoplanin 118
Temperature 106
   management 86
Tension pneumothorax 80
Terbutaline 83, 152
   nebulizer 83
Tetany 42
Tetralogy of Fallot 132, 133*f*
Thermodilution 19
Thermometer 2
Thiocyanate 99
Thoracic duct ligation 82
Thrombocytopenia 48, 99
Ticarcillin clavulanate 119
Ticloplanin 161
Tissue
   hypoperfusion 20
   plasminogen activator 165
Tonoferon 157
Total anomalous pulmonary venous connection 12, 131
Total parenteral nutrition 76, 90, 165
   complications of 77
Trace elements 77
Tracheomalacia 79
Tracheostomy 108
   care 108

tube 110, 113
    care of 109
    cuffed 109
    fenestrated 110
Tramadol 157
Tranexamic acid 47
Transfusion therapy 45
Transthoracic thoracic pacemaker 64
Trauma 11
    surgical 61
Tremor 101
Triclofos 156
Tricuspid
    atresia 58
    insufficiency 26
    stenosis 11
Triglycerides 77
Trimethoprim 119
Truncus arteriosus 134, 134f
Tubes, removal of 70
Tumor, atrial 58

U

Upper airways obstructions 79
Upper gastrointestinal bleed 84
Urinalysis 37
Urinary catheter 6
    care of 106
Urinary sodium 88
Urine
    collection system 2
    osmolarity 88
    output 17, 22

V

Vagal maneuvers 57
Vagal tone, high-level of 61
Valve
    repair 103
    stenosis, persistent 16
Valvuloplasty 137
Vancomycin 117-119, 161
Vascular resistance, systemic 12, 17
Vasoconstriction, peripheral 99
Vasodilatation 114
    pulmonary 98
    venous 99
Vasodilators 99, 148
Vasopressin 100
Vecuronium 30, 95
Velocity time integral method 19
Ventilation 53, 133, 142
    alveolar 15
    dead space 15
    high-frequency oscillation 30
    noninvasive 131
    setting up volume-controlled 29
Ventilator 2, 4, 29
    connections 6
    setting 29
    time-cycled 28
Ventricular
    dysfunction 22
    fibrillation 54, 60, 62
    premature beat 56, 59
    rate 56, 57, 63
    septal defect 54, 103, 129, 130
        murmur 18
    synchronous pacing 67
    tachycardia 54, 60, 62
Ventriculotomy 133
    incisions 16
Verapamil 57
Vertigo 101
Vital signs 4
Vitamin 77
Vocal cord
    dysfunction 79
    paralysis, permanent left 79
Volume controlled syndronized intermittent mandatory ventilation 29
Vomiting 40, 41, 101
von Willebrand's disease 51
von Willebrand's factor 51
V-wave 11

W

Warfarin sodium 153
Weaning 31, 34
Wheeze 83
White blood cell counts, regular 114
Wolff-Parkinson-White syndrome 59

X

X-descent 11
X-ray, abdominal 84

Y

Y-descent 11
Yersinia enterocolitica 119

Z

Zosyn 161

EU GSPR Authorised Reprsentative
Logos Europe, 9 rue Nicolas Poussin
1700, La Rochelle, France
Phone: +33 (0) 6 67 93 73 78
E-mail: contact@logoseurope.eu

www.ingramcontent.com/pod-product-compliance
Ingram Content Group UK Ltd.
Pitfield, Milton Keynes, MK11 3LW, UK
UKHW021828140426
5217IPUK00016B/1252